# Understanding Health Inequalities
# in Aotearoa New Zealand

# Understanding Health Inequalities in Aotearoa New Zealand

Edited by
Kevin Dew and Anna Matheson

Otago University Press

OTAGO

Published by Otago University Press
PO Box 56/Level 1, 398 Cumberland Street, Dunedin, New Zealand
Fax: 64 3 479 8385
Email: university.press@otago.ac.nz
Website: www.otago.ac.nz/press

First published 2008
Copyright © Kevin Dew and Anna Matheson 2008
ISBN 978 1 877372 59 9

Book and cover design by Fiona Moffat
Printed in New Zealand by Astra Print Ltd, Wellington

# Contents

# Acknowledgements

The idea for this book was born out of a conference titled *Health Inequalities and Need: Pathways to Interventions* held at Te Papa Tongarewa in Wellington on 27 August 2004. The editors were on the organising committee for this conference but would like to thank others on that committee: Vonda Tuamata, Ian Prior, Win Bennett, Tony Blakely, Peter Crampton, Philippa Howden-Chapman, Tim Rochford, Louise Signal and Keitha Small, and Gay Keating for her support. We would also like to thank the following organisations for providing funding for that conference: the Health Research Council of New Zealand, the Social Policy Evaluation and Research Committee, and Capital and Coast District Health Board. We would also like to thank speakers who were not able to contribute to this book: Papaarangi Reid, Deborah Ryan, Tony Blakely and David Slack, and to thank Sir Paul Reeves for his generosity in chairing the conference.

Thanks also to the Department of Public Health at the Wellington School of Medicine and Health Sciences for providing the time and space to work on this project and the intellectual environment for engaging with issues discussed in this book. A special thank you to all the contributors to this book for their commitment and responsiveness. They come from a range of disciplines and backgrounds, and for the editors this has been both a challenge and a pleasure.

KEVIN DEW AND ANNA MATHESON
*Wellington, February 2008*

# 1. Health, justice and politics

Anna Matheson and Kevin Dew

**A** baby boy born in Swaziland today can expect to reach the age of 36, a baby boy born in Japan can expect to reach the age of 79 (World Health Organization 2006). Such are the extremes of health inequalities on a global scale. Closer to home, the life expectancy of a new-born baby boy in one of the most deprived areas in Aotearoa New Zealand is nine years less than that of a baby boy born in one of the least deprived areas (see Hill, Chapter 3 of this book). Māori aged between 45 and 64 are three times more likely to die than others in this age group in Aotearoa New Zealand (see Robson, Chapter 2). Genetics, lifestyle choices, and technological developments do not explain the extent of such differences. These health inequalities are profoundly shaped by the way we organise society, as well as by our history and our place in the world.

Health inequalities are the unequal distribution of health outcomes within and between populations. Much work has been done in recent years to describe health inequalities and attempt to understand not just causes of specific health outcomes for populations but also how and why health inequalities arise in complex social systems. In societies like Aotearoa New Zealand, health inequalities have been associated with an array of social factors, the most consistently interrogated being class or socio-economic status, gender, ethnicity, and geographical location (Gray 2006). How these social factors impact on health depends on how they interact with each other, as well as the particular historical moment and its specific alignment of politics, economics, culture, and social practices. Because of this complexity simple, quick-fix solutions to health inequalities are unlikely to be found.

The content of this book reflects this complexity. We have taken account of the different ways in which people might have experienced, thought about, and analysed health inequalities. As a result, the chapters are diverse, both in the detail of description and analysis, and in the style of writing. The book takes the view that in order to understand this complexity and its outcomes, it is crucial to consider the role of relationships: not merely acknowledging that relationships exist, but investigating their qualitative nature; in other words, looking at how meaningful connections between individuals, between language, between social environments, between levels of social organisation, between the present and the past, and between ways of thinking about and expressing ideas are made.

The first part of the book (Chapters 1–4) offers a picture of health inequalities in New Zealand. The second part (Chapters 5–9) provides ways of understanding health inequalities. The third (Chapters 10–13) explores practical efforts to alter these trends and reduce health inequalities, and the fourth and final part (Chapters 14–15) offers insights into the experiences of those who deliver health services at the coalface. The contributors come from a variety of disciplines and perspectives including community leaders and workers, policy-makers and implementers, epidemiologists, public health researchers, economists, sociologists, historians, and medical professionals.

Before briefly outlining the chapters, we offer the following context for this interest in and attention to health inequalities in New Zealand.

## The politics of inequality

The notion of health inequalities has had a chequered and politically charged recent history within Aotearoa New Zealand. The turbulent decades of the 1980s and 1990s saw vigorous and swift changes to economic and social policy. This opening up of the economy, which involved substantial welfare reforms and a move towards 'efficiency' in the public sector, was viewed by many commentators as responsible for increasing social inequality in New Zealand (for example, Peters 1997; Roper 2005). Helen Clark's Labour-led government came into power in 1999 on a platform of ideas of social inclusion, an acknowledgement of the role and significance of the community or 'third sector', and of the injustice of social inequality (Craig & Porter 2005).

In response to these concerns about increasing social inequalities, explicit policies were developed. The ways in which these policies have been received, altered, abandoned, and revived illustrate the politically charged nature of the topic of social and health inequalities. Early in its first term, Labour's social policies unabashedly targeted social and economic inequalities; they had descriptive labels such as 'Closing the Gaps' and 'Treaty-based'. The gaps that were to be closed were inequalities in health and social outcomes between different socio-economic groups, but these policies also became strongly identified with addressing the disparities between Pākehā and Māori. The inequalities agenda revalidated targeting Māori specifically, in order to redress historical issues associated with colonisation and honouring the intent of the Treaty of Waitangi.

As Belgrave discusses (Chapter 5), 'Closing the Gaps' suffered from political pressure, and the rhetoric was subsequently abandoned. However, the government's stated commitment to reducing inequalities (Ministry of Social Policy 2001) continued through more specific and less politically charged areas; for example, it was the subject of a number of official Ministry of Health publications, and District Health Boards have a statutory requirement to reduce health inequalities (Ministry of Health 2002).

A watershed event in the health inequalities debate in Aotearoa New Zealand occurred on 27 January 2004 when Don Brash, then leader of a weakened National Party, gave an address, known as the Orewa speech, to the Orewa Rotary Club. In this speech he claimed that government funding for health (as well as education) was influenced by the ethnicity of the recipient – and not need. He claimed that this was racially divisive and that a National government would remove funding based on ethnicity. As Jon Johansson argues: 'He talks, almost absurdly given the disparity between Māori and Pākehā outcomes on any number of social indicators, of a New Zealand where "the minority has a birthright to the upper hand"' (Johansson 2004: 112). The immediate consequence of this speech was that the National Party rose 17 points in opinion polls, with the greatest support coming from men and blue-collar workers (Johansson 2004). Johansson goes on to say:

> The fact that Brash's evidence for 'privilege' was frequently anecdotal and remarkably thin when compared to every social indicator reveals how emotion, when stimulated, can swamp reason, especially when saliency about race issues is high (Johansson 2004: 115).

The longer-term consequences of Brash's speech are harder to quantify but concern was expressed that this overly simplified view of how to address health inequalities could have untoward consequences for a range of programmes. This book contributes to this debate and advocates reason, not emotion, as the best way to understand and address health inequalities.

This political manoeuvring also touched on one of the more substantive debates around understanding inequalities – individual versus social causes of inequality. The National Party rhetoric of 'all New Zealanders' gave the impression of collectivity while individual need gave the impression of equity. But, as many contributors to this book discuss, understanding health inequalities requires an understanding that population 'need' is different to individual 'need'. The powerful social forces that have an impact on health status are beyond the influence of individuals.

## Health inequalities in New Zealand
*... causes of individual cases are not the same as the causes of overall incidence* (Geoffrey Rose cited in Evans 2002: 6)

The disciplines of epidemiology and social epidemiology have provided an increasingly rich description of health inequalities. In turn, a great deal of thought has gone into trying to understand why certain patterns emerge. Whereas epidemiology has traditionally focused on how and from where infectious diseases spread, social epidemiology explores the patterning of health outcomes through their association with social characteristics such as income, gender and ethnicity in an attempt to find the causes of these differences between groups.

On a global scale there is an enormous variation in life expectancy between different countries and world regions (World Health Organization 2006). Within countries, the situation is similar, although the shape of inequalities varies given local conditions such as history, economy, and social structure. In New Zealand, the picture of inequality has become more vivid over the past 10 years with a number of initiatives mapping, measuring, and describing it.

As the incident described in the previous section suggests, the notions of 'race' and 'ethnicity' hold an important and politically charged place in the New Zealand context. Indeed, 'ethnicity', particularly as it applies to Māori, is an important and well-researched measure in New Zealand. In Chapter 2, Bridget Robson provides an overview of the pattern of difference in health outcomes for Māori and non-Māori, with a focus on the relationship between these patterns and aspects of the economy. Robson clearly demonstrates the need to understand our history in order to understand its enduring consequences on health outcomes, arguing that health justice and social justice are inextricably interwoven. Chris Cunningham, in Chapter 4, takes an intra-ethnic view of the different life experiences and issues related to health within the Māori population. He notes that better knowledge of the diverse experiences of Māori should inform interventions to reduce inequalities, in relation to both 'by Māori for Māori' services and mainstream services.

In Chapter 3, Sarah Hill gives an overview of the history and evidence of measuring and describing health inequalities from the perspective of social epidemiology in New Zealand. This chapter strongly emphasises the substantial influence that social factors have on health outcomes and health inequality. By tracing changes over time, Hill shows that the patterns of health inequalities are not fixed and immutable, suggesting that with will and determination, alongside better understanding of both the underlying mechanisms that cause health inequality and the interventions that can redress them, a more equitable society is achievable.

It should be noted that the measurement of health inequalities is neither simple nor straightforward. To develop measures that allow comparisons between people or groups, a numerical measure of 'health' and a numerical measure of relevant social factors need to be found. For health, proxy measures have to be used, such as rates of mortality or life expectancy. Rates of morbidity (or disease and injury) can also be used. Some social factors can be relatively easily determined, such as age or gender. It is, however, much more difficult to find good measures of such things as social class or even ethnicity. Sarah Hill notes changes in measurement of social class in her chapter, and Chris Cunningham explores some aspects of measuring ethnicity. Nevertheless it should be noted that whichever solution is found to measure particular social factors, they are persistently and consistently related to inequalities in health.

Another issue often raised when considering the relationship of social factors to health inequalities is: what is the cause and what is the effect? To illustrate, if we take income as a proxy measure for social class, we could ask: are people poor because they are ill or have a disability and therefore have a reduced earning capacity? It might be assumed that people are in lower social classes because they are sicker than others, not because the social class itself has had an impact on their health. This is known as the selective mobility hypothesis. Sick people who may have been well off previously may move down the social scale as their earning capacity drops, and sick people who are already poor are less able to move up the scale. Alternatively, are people ill and do they have disabilities because of their level of deprivation and their low income?

In order to find out which is the dominant effect, studies have to be carried out over a long time to track people in relation to their income and health status. The international literature does not support the selective mobility hypothesis as an explanation for the relationship between health and income. Indeed, living on a consistently low income predicts an increased risk of premature death. When initial health status is taken into account, the relationship still holds (O'Dea & Howden-Chapman 2000). In other words, people are not poor because they are sick; they are sick because they are poor.

## Understanding health inequalities

To enhance our understanding of the production and reproduction of health inequalities it is necessary to draw on insights from a range of disciplines and to consider a variety of factors and influences. Within social epidemiology, a virulent debate has taken place around income inequality and the evidence that there is an income gradient in health outcomes. The two competing arguments that have often polarised this debate are that this gradient is either caused by the lack of access to material assets or that it is caused by 'psycho-social' factors (see Chapter 7 for Brian Easton's discussion on this issue). The first of these arguments suggests that unequal access to material factors such as good nutrition, decent housing, health care, and other things that money can buy has an impact on the health of individuals.

The psycho-social argument has been given credence by a famous research programme studying the stress effects of hierarchy, known as the Whitehall study (Brunner & Marmot 1999). This programme studied 17,000 British civil servants. It found that there was a relationship between the employment grade in the civil service and health-related psycho-social factors. These factors included low control over work, a lack of variety in work, and a lack of social contact. The researchers found that there were metabolic changes associated with a person's position in the workplace hierarchy, including changes in blood glucose levels and blood-clotting mechanisms. The research supports the view that long-term exposure to psycho-social stresses in the workplace may lead to increased risk of conditions such as heart disease and diabetes. Although these studies have been limited to workplaces, the mechanisms affecting health could apply to the general population. Wherever people experience stress related to rigid hierarchies and a lack of control over their actions, adverse health effects might follow. The psycho-social argument has led to discussion of the influence of social hierarchy and the implication that relative inequality (not just absolute inequality, where material factors are most influential) might affect health outcomes.

Both the materialist and psycho-social arguments focus on our immediate environment. But to deepen our understanding, it is necessary to look at the context in which health services are delivered and social practices occur. Michael Belgrave, in Chapter 5, lends an historian's perspective. He argues that past developments in health and social policies impact on the present shape of these policies, and an understanding of the past means that discussions of present constraints and possibilities will be better informed. In Chapter 6, Tim McCreanor explores the impact that communication and ways of talking have on creating and maintaining social order, and how the way in which we talk about ethnicity and race (or the discourses we use) plays an important part in the occurrence and persistence of discrimination, which in turn impacts upon health.

Chapters 7 and 8 explore the relationship between income, poverty, policy, and health. Brian Easton argues that both the material and psycho-social hypotheses are needed to explain some of the changes in the relationship between health outcomes and income in recent decades in Aotearoa New Zealand. He argues that any policy changes should be audited to determine the stress they will generate, and so broaden the focus beyond material change. Susan St John reflects on the complex issue of child poverty, noting that the relative economic position of the poorest children in Aotearoa continues to deteriorate and that this has major implications, not only for the immediate health status of these children but also for their long-term health outcomes. The final chapter in part two, by John Forman, looks at a particular group that tends to be left out of most debates about health inequalities – those who suffer from rare disorders. Forman argues that in the struggle over scarce resources between community, primary care, and clinical services this significant group is left out. Forman's chapter is a call to broaden the debate and he provides a number of principles that should be considered in this process.

## Intervening to reduce health inequalities

Although we are gaining an increasingly nuanced picture of health inequalities and engaging in more sophisticated debates that extend our understanding of the causes, there has until quite recently been less concentration on the practice of intervening to reduce these inequalities. Part of this neglect seems to lie in the complexities of the interactions that lead to health inequalities and in the complexities of moving from evidence to action.

The notion of 'health inequalities' helps shape how we should think about interventions, as it depicts outcomes at a broad system level. Rather than viewing intervention narrowly, as a one-off action where outcomes are evaluated at the site of intervention, this broader view sees interventions as a process that attempts to bring about change.

Part of the challenge here is that there is very little empirical evidence from activities which have an explicit focus on reducing health inequalities either in terms of effectiveness or in terms of the theories of intervention. Where there is, the quantitative evidence of effectiveness is often equivocal, with calls for greater concentration within the literature on understanding more about the connection between individuals and societal structures, as well as greater understanding of social complexity generally (Sorensen *et al*. 1998; Bauld *et al*. 2005). The literature and evidence show that the understanding of certain aspects of interventions such as the local context, the role of relationships, the role of organisations, issues of trust and power, and the capacity to change are critical to gaining insight into intervention success and having more realistic expectations of what outcomes can be achieved (Bauld *et al*. 2005).

In Chapter 10, Peter Crampton and Jan Foley illuminate the way in which primary health care services are funded. He explores the variety of ways in which services have been and could be funded, spelling out the rationale for the current funding formulas. He concludes that although Aotearoa New Zealand has made some progress in attempting to use funding formulas to reduce inequalities, more could be done. The issue of health service funding is an important one to understand as there has been a great deal of debate about how services are funded and who might be privileged, without very much knowledge about the actual processes.

In Chapter 11, Julia Carr and Lee Tan explore the relationship between primary care services and attempts to reduce inequalities, and discuss the development of the Primary Health Care Strategy and its implementation. This strategy led to the development of Primary Health Organisations (PHOs), which are required to work with communities and other agencies to address significant primary care and other population health issues. Carr and Tan describe a range of activities undertaken by PHOs to reduce inequalities, but they also note the complex issues that face PHOs. They suggest that although new structures are important in fostering change, what is required is a more fundamental shift in thinking so that there is a greater local role in decision-making and ownership.

Philippa Howden-Chapman and Sarah Bierre provide insights into reducing health inequalities through housing interventions. Their chapter notes the relationship between housing and health inequalities, and describes a number of interventions to improve housing; it also looks at how research can facilitate better assessments of housing's impact on health outcomes. Howden-Chapman and Bierre argue that housing is a very appropriate site for public health interventions aimed at reducing inequalities. The last chapter in this section, from Louise Signal, looks at interventions that have been developed to orient the health sector itself to the issue of health inequalities, and how these can be reduced, maintained or exacerbated by work in the health sector. The 'health sector' here refers to the whole range of people who work in the health area, from policy-makers to those delivering the huge range of health services available, including those working in government ministries, health provider organisations, and non-governmental organisations.

In the final part of this book we hear the voices of those who work at the coalface of health services delivery – those who are actively engaged in reducing health inequalities. Olivia James provides a vivid description of the situation in Otara that led to the formation of Otara Health Inc., a health promotion organisation. Her chapter provides an account of the difficulties faced in developing an organisation that did not fit the funders' mould, and of the successes that allowed the organisation to survive and develop. For James, the Otara story shows how a community that is seen as disadvantaged can develop local solutions to local problems. Win Bennett, Eugene Ryder, Maude Governor, Kathy James, Maggie Simcox, and Leanne Ormsby conclude part four with lucid accounts of what is required to improve the health of those who do not readily access mainstream health services. One of the conclusions drawn from these stories is that policy-makers need to take more seriously the role of relationships at the community level, putting less emphasis on accountability and more on trust.

In sum, although this book is arranged in a logical order, starting with a picture of inequalities, then moving on to an understanding of their production and reproduction, then to interventions and finally to the experience of those who work with those most affected by health inequalities, the reality is not so linear. An understanding of the relationships between all these parts of the picture is needed, together with a reminder that policies, when implemented, have a real impact on people's lives.

This book has been a labour of love on the part of the editors and contributors. The chapters in this book represent the situation at a particular point in time. The picture of health inequalities and the policy responses are not static but are ever-changing. Many of the specific issues mentioned may quickly change in character – but the underlying issues that are discussed are enduring. For all of us, health inequalities, and social inequalities generally, are an issue of great importance that cannot be left to politicians looking to improve their standing in the opinion polls. It is hoped that this collection of essays will play some part in raising the level of debate about social and health inequalities in Aotearoa New Zealand, support the good work that is already being done, and provide the motivation for much more desperately needed work.

# Part One
Ethnic and Socio-economic
Inequalities in Health

# 2. What is driving the disparities?

Bridget Robson

Systematic disparities in health outcomes between the Māori and non-Māori populations of Aotearoa New Zealand have persisted for far too long. This chapter describes some of the major disparities in health outcomes between Māori and non-Māori, and then explores some of the reasons for the persistence of these disparities. A few examples are chosen to illustrate the complex relationship between the economy and Māori health, namely the labour market, tobacco policy, and child poverty. In the process, a host of factors that impact negatively on Māori health, such as the history of colonialism, the effects of racism and the outcomes of poverty are touched on. The chapter starts from an understanding that disparities in health are the result of the differential distribution of economic and social determinants of health and seeks to understand the drivers of this unequal distribution between Māori and non-Māori.

To discuss economic determinants and health it is also necessary to discuss the rights enshrined in the Treaty of Waitangi and breaches of these rights, human rights, indigenous peoples' rights, and ethical obligations. Many indigenous nations are struggling with the realities that underpin health statistics and reflect disparities in health outcomes. The struggles of these peoples resound with stories of resistance, consistent and ongoing reaffirmation and assertion of rights, and renewal of relationships with the environment, tūpuna, and the generations to come.

There is a strong driving force among Māori for economic, educational, social, cultural, and health development. 'By Māori for Māori' providers in education, health, and social services are growing in number and size. Many are providing services for all New Zealanders. Māori-owned and -operated businesses are increasing, and the demand for education is flourishing as Māori-controlled education institutions provide effective learning environments for all age-groups. Whānau, hapū, iwi, and other Māori collectives are building strategies for positive long-term development.

However, Māori-led services still only receive a tiny fraction of government funding, limiting the access of many Māori to such services and perpetuating structural inequalities by forcing Māori initiatives to operate on inadequate funding. At the same time, discrimination in education and the labour market not only creates powerful restraints and restrictions on Māori access to the health and social benefits that are available to non-Māori, but also hinders Māori from maximising the opportunities provided by Māori initiatives.

Health justice and economic justice are closely intertwined. Decades of untenable and increasing disparities in longevity in Aotearoa have accompanied an increasingly inequitable and unjust distribution of the fruits of the nation's economy. Recent struggles concerning title to the seabed and foreshore, and the commercial and political interests being served in these struggles, provide a stark reminder that colonialism is a continuous force that has been impacting on Māori economy and health since the early nineteenth century. Indeed, the history of this impact on Māori echoes the experience of other indigenous nations in settler-colonial lands throughout the world.

## Health trends

Recent research shows that during the late 1980s and 1990s disparities between Māori and non-Māori increased significantly as measured by a number of key health indicators: life expectancy, cancer mortality, and cardiovascular rates (Ajwani *et al*. 2003). The difference in life expectancy between Māori and non-Māori grew to 10 years. Research also shows some disturbing trends in the provision of health services: for example, despite high mortality from heart disease among Māori and Pacific peoples, cardiac interventions were most frequently received by non-Māori, non-Pacific people (Tukuitonga & Bindman 2002).

The impact of colonial settlement on Māori health is well established. Disease, conflict and dispossession led to a decline in the Māori population by one-third or more during the late nineteenth century. The twentieth century witnessed a regeneration of the Māori population and a rapid narrowing of the life-expectancy gap between Māori and non-Māori during the three decades after World War II (Pool 1991; Pōmare *et al*. 1995).

From the mid-1980s, however, research shows a new and significant widening of the disparities in Māori and non-Māori life expectancy (Ajwani *et al* 2003). Figure 2.1 shows, in the two decades from 1980 to 2000, non-Māori life expectancy at birth increased at a faster rate than at any time since World War II, while the increase for Māori was minimal.

Mortality rates declined for non-Māori across all age groups, while remaining relatively static for Māori. Thus mortality gaps widened in both sexes and in each age group. The largest disparities were evident in the 45–64 year age groups, among whom Māori rates of all-cause mortality were three times those of non-Māori, non-Pacific in 1996–9 (Figure 2.2).

Cardiovascular disease, cancer, respiratory disease, and injury were the major causes of death for both Māori and non-Māori. Cancer mortality decreased steadily among non-Māori and non-Pacific populations but actually increased for Māori (Figure 2.3).

Cardiovascular mortality decreased for both Māori and non-Māori, but to a lesser extent for Māori (Figure 2.4). By 1996–9 Māori males had three times

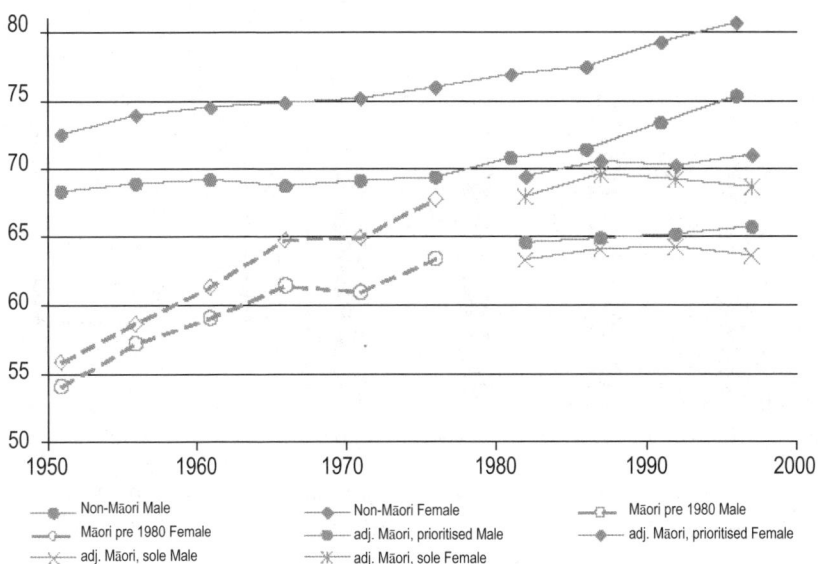

*Figure 2.1: Māori and non-Māori life expectancy at birth by gender, 1950–2000. (Source: Ajwani et al. 2003)*

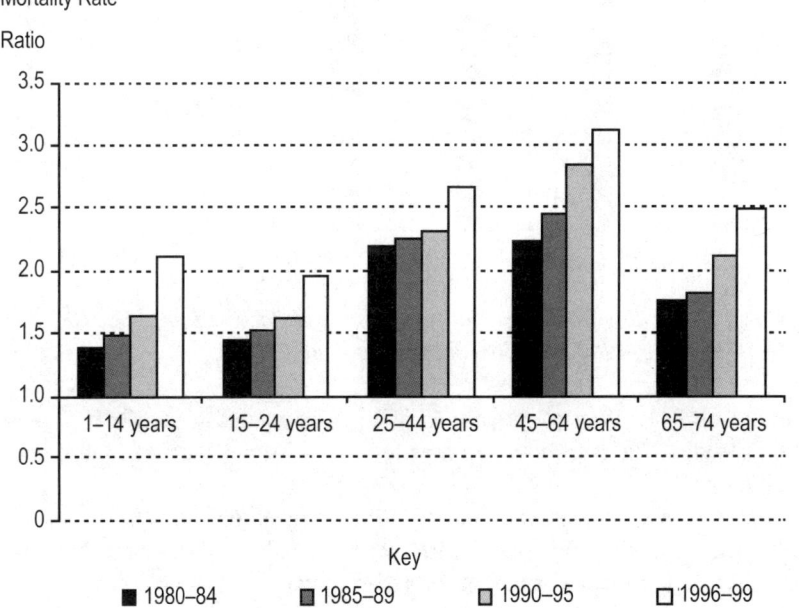

*Figure 2.2: Māori/non-Māori non-Pacific mortality rate ratios by age group 1980–99. (Source: Ajwani et al. 2003)*

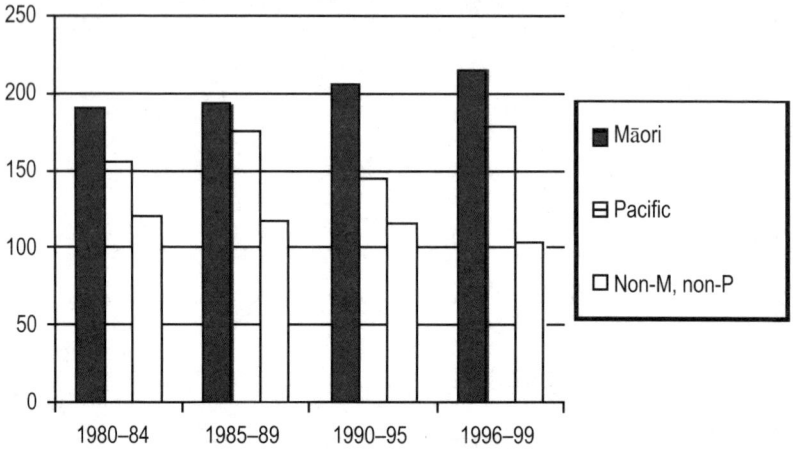

*Figure 2.3: Cancer mortality, age-sex standardised rates per 100,000, ages 1–74 years, 1980–99. (Source: Ajwani et al. 2003)*

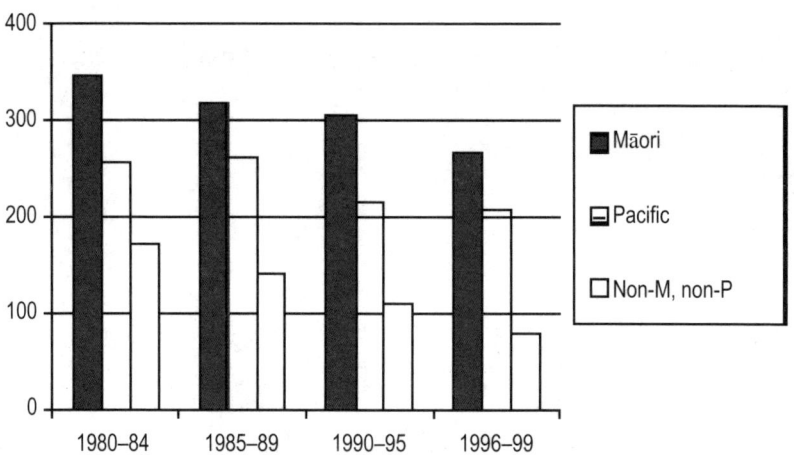

*Figure 2.4: Cardiovascular mortality, age-sex standardised rates per 100,000, ages 1–74 years, 1980–99. (Source: Ajwani et al. 2003)*

the rate of death from cardiovascular disease compared to non-Māori, non-Pacific males. The rate for Māori females was 4.2 times the non-Māori, non-Pacific rate.

In terms of cardiovascular deaths, mortality rates for stroke decreased for both Māori and non-Māori, but in 1996–9 Māori males had twice the mortality rate of non-Māori males, and that for Māori females was three times the non-Māori rate. Gaps widened for deaths from ischaemic heart disease, as non-Māori rates decreased substantially over the twenty-year period, but the decline for Māori was less, especially among Māori males. Despite the higher mortality

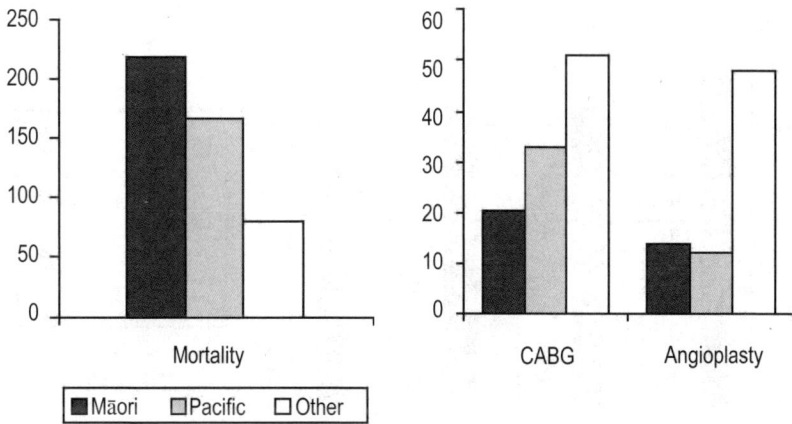

*Figure 2.5: Ischaemic heart disease mortality 1996–9 and rates of publicly funded coronary artery bypass and graft and angioplasty 1990–9. Age-standardised rates[1] per 100,000 for Māori, Pacific and other males. (Source: Ajwani et al. 2003; Tukuitonga & Bindman 2002)*

from heart disease among Māori and Pacific peoples, cardiac interventions were most frequently received by non-Māori non-Pacific people during this period (Tukuitonga & Bindman 2002). Figure 2.5 shows male mortality rates for 1996–9 compared with publicly funded cardiac interventions in 1990–9. These patterns held, even when controlling for gender, age and deprivation (Westbrooke *et al.* 2000).

Deaths from unintentional injury decreased among Māori and non-Māori between 1980–4 and 1996–9. However, the rate for Māori remained twice as high as that of non-Māori (Figure 2.6). Road traffic crashes were the main cause of death from unintentional injury (Ajwani *et al.* 2003).

Rates of suicide in the 15–24 and 25–44 age groups were previously lower among Māori than non-Māori. However, Māori rates of youth suicide (especially among males) accelerated during the 1980s. Indeed, by 1996–9, Māori rates (among both males and females) were twice those of non-Māori. Figure 2.7 shows suicide rates for males aged 15–24 years. Similar increases occurred among Māori aged 25–44 years, although the rates were lower in that age group. Female rates were about a third of male rates (Ajwani *et al.* 2003). Male youth suicide rates may be starting to decline, but rates remain higher among Māori than non-Māori (NZHIS 2004). Among young females, the Māori rate of hospital admissions for intentional self-harm is about a fifth lower than the rate for non-Māori. Among young males, the rate for Māori is about a fifth higher than for non-Māori (NZHIS 2004).

Trends in infant deaths were similar to those for other age groups, with decreases among such deaths for both Māori and non-Māori over the 20-year period. However, because the decrease was much greater for non-Māori

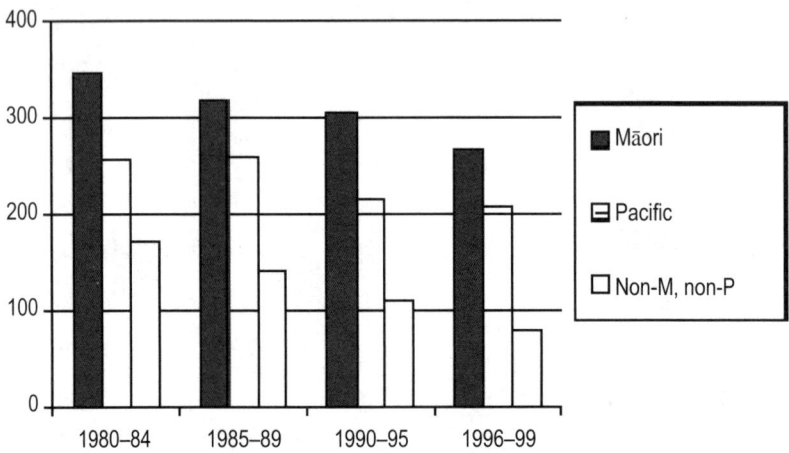

*Figure 2.6: Unintentional injury mortality 1980–99. Age-sex standardised rates per 100,000. (Source: Ajwani et al. 2003)*

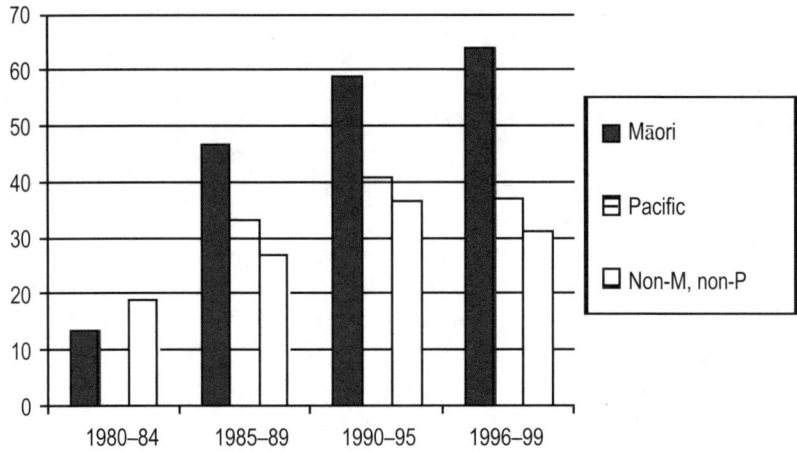

*Figure 2.7: Suicide rates per 100,000 among males aged 15–24 years, 1980–99. (Source: Ajwani et al. 2003)*

infants than for Māori infants, disparities have widened considerably during this period. Infant deaths were twice as common among Māori babies (9.2 per 1000 live births) than non-Māori babies (4.6 per 1000 live births) in 1999. Sudden Infant Death Syndrome (SIDS) is the main contributor to this trend of increasing disparity, as the SIDS prevention campaign was more effective for non-Māori than for Māori (Tipene-Leach *et al.* 2000).

In summary, during the 1980s and 1990s mortality decreased steadily among non-Māori but only minimally among Māori. Cancer mortality actually increased for Māori, while it decreased for Pākehā. Heart disease mortality declined rapidly among Pākehā, but slowly among Māori. Unintentional injury deaths declined for both groups, but the gap did not close. Youth suicide rates increased among both Māori and non-Māori, but at a much faster rate among Māori. The gap in life expectancy between Māori and non-Māori increased to 10 years. Evidence that disparities are increasing underscores the imperative for action to eliminate ethnic inequalities in health. In order to determine what action to take, a better understanding of what underlies these differences and why they are so enduring is needed. The following sections provide examples that help illuminate some of the reasons for the existence and persistence of health disparities between Māori and non-Māori. These examples are the labour market, tobacco consumption, and child poverty.

## Labour market segregation and health disparities

Income and wealth are strong predictors of health, affecting access to healthy environments and living conditions, education, housing, and timely, effective health care. Levels of home ownership, property ownership, and income-producing assets are lower among Māori than among non-Māori (Te Puni Kōkiri 2000). In addition, lower equivalent income levels limit the ability of Māori families to accumulate wealth out of current income. Market income (wages and salary) is therefore the most common source of income for Māori, and thus the labour market is a vital structural determinant of Māori health and disparities.

A number of issues in the labour market have led to Māori being disadvantaged and have thus contributed to the disparities described above. Key issues include differences in occupational injury deaths, the different distribution of Māori and non-Māori across occupational classes, and discrimination in the labour market.

A study of work-related fatal injury during 1985–94 found a significantly higher crude risk of death among Māori male workers than among non-Māori male workers aged 15–84 years (McCracken *et al.* 2001). The study found that the overall difference in rates of work-related fatal injury was likely to be due to contrasting employment patterns between Māori and non-Māori workforces. In more dangerous forms of employment, there was a higher concentration of Māori than non-Māori workers. Furthermore, the study revealed a significant downward trend in occupational fatality rates for non-Māori over the decade, but no corresponding decrease in Māori rates.

Strong occupational class gradients in premature mortality among Māori and non-Māori men aged 15–64 years were observed during the 1970s and 1980s (Pearce *et al.* 1984; Smith & Pearce 1984; Pearce *et al.* 1993). In both decades, Māori mortality rates per occupational level were higher than non-Māori rates.

The occupational class gradient was steeper for deaths from 'amenable' causes. Within each occupational group, Māori men had a higher risk of death than non-Māori (more than 3.5 times higher) producing a rate 5.8 times higher overall, reducing to 4.8 when controlled for occupational class. These causes of death are considered largely avoidable given appropriate medical intervention.[2] Although it is recognised that death is the final event in a complex chain that includes environmental, lifestyle, and socio-economic processes, as well as preventive and curative health care (Nolte & McKee 2003), these findings signal that the New Zealand health services appear to be meeting Pākehā health needs ahead of serious Māori health needs.

Discrimination in the labour market occurs at a number of different points, namely job discrimination, occupational segregation, and wage discrimination. This leads to structural inequalities in New Zealand's labour market favouring Pākehā and constraining Māori development. The June 2001 Income Survey showed that Māori men and women earned on average 80.5 per cent of the hourly pay earned by Pākehā men and women (Minitatanga mō ngā Wāhine 2002).

Māori men earned on average 76 per cent of the average hourly earnings of Pākehā men, and 92.3 per cent of the average hourly pay earned by Pākehā women. Māori women earned on average 70.6 per cent of the average hourly pay earned by Pākehā men, 85.6 per cent of the average hourly pay earned by Pākehā women, and 92.8 per cent of the average hourly pay earned by Māori men.

This data shows that the ethnicity pay gap in New Zealand is greater than the gender pay gap, as Māori men earn less than Pākehā women. However, the figures also show that Māori women experience both a gender and an ethnicity pay gap (Minitatanga mō ngā Wāhine 2002).

Discrimination could potentially operate at four main points in an individual's labour-market experience (Sutherland & Alexander 2002; Alexander *et al.* 2003): first, in the pre-labour market; then, having entered the labour market, in obtaining work (job discrimination); third, in gaining a particular type of work (occupational segregation), and finally in the wages paid for a particular type of work (wage discrimination).

The development of a New Zealand socio-economic index of occupational status (Davis *et al.* 1997) provided evidence that New Zealand society assigns a higher value to Pākehā-dominated occupations than to Māori-dominated occupations. Occupational segregation may thus operate not only to exclude Māori (and also women) from higher 'status' positions, but also to maintain higher levels of reward for occupations that are dominated by Pākehā (and also by males).

Significant occupational segregation in the New Zealand labour market was found by Sutherland and Alexander (2002), with Māori consistently under-represented in the two highest occupational levels and over-represented in the two lowest levels, even after taking education and other productivity characteristics into account. Wage discrimination was also found – mostly due to underpayment of Māori within occupational classes and some overpayment of Pākehā. Thus between 29.3 per cent and 47.7 per cent of the Pākehā/Māori wage differential was found to be attributable to some form of discrimination, with both underpayment of Māori within occupational classes and job discrimination evident.

This occupational segregation is an important factor in explaining the particularly severe impact on Māori health during times of economic upheaval. The uneven impact of New Zealand's economic restructuring in the 1980s was predicted by Māori leaders who warned against policies that would 'make Māori the "shock absorbers in the economy" through hitting those at the bottom of the economic ladder hardest during poor times, while rewarding those at the top of the economic ladder during good times' (Pōmare et al. 1995: 149). The abrupt widening of the life expectancy gap since the mid-1980s indicates the depth of the impact on Māori health. Conversely, the acceleration in Pākehā life expectancy during this period, which included a serious economic recession, points to the existence of what Bhattacharyya and colleagues term the 'wages of whiteness' in Aotearoa (Bhattacharyya et al. 2002). Carlson argues that the racialisation of the American labour force enabled many white Americans to cushion themselves from the full effects of economic restructuring. He warns that 'conservative and rightist politics in the years ahead are thus likely to be based on a tacit appeal to maintaining white economic privilege in the face of massive economic shifts' (1997: 145).

United States psychologists Samuel Gaertner, John Dovidio, and colleagues have a substantial programme of research on reducing intergroup bias. It focuses on how overt racism has evolved into more subtle and insidious forms than the traditional forms of discrimination, practised unintentionally by liberal white Americans who believe they are not prejudiced against blacks and hold genuinely egalitarian values. Their research has identified what they describe as 'aversive racism' – characterised more by 'pro-white (pro-ingroup)' bias rather than 'anti-black (anti-outgroup)' attitudes (Gaertner et al. 1997). Aversive racism produces an emotional reaction that is 'not one of overt dislike or hostility, but rather one of anxiety or discomfort', which means that inter-ethnic interaction is avoided (Dovidio 1997: 378). Those influenced by 'aversive racism' consciously endorse egalitarian values and therefore try not to behave in overtly negative ways (as such behaviour would threaten their self-image as unbiased). However, their bias is frequently expressed indirectly 'by favouring whites rather than discriminating against blacks and members of other minority groups' (Dovidio 1997: 378).

Aversive racism may be enacted through providing special favours, support, mentoring or promotion opportunities to people with backgrounds similar to their own. The higher proportion of Pākehā in managerial occupations and the higher social status assigned to Pākehā male-dominated occupations (Davis et al. 1997) where there is more power to mentor, promote, hire, and fire individuals indicates there is ample scope for aversive racism to maintain or even to increase the current occupational segregation favouring Pākehā.

# Tobacco consumption and its
# disproportionate impact on Māori

Tobacco is a major cause of preventable death in Aotearoa. Tobacco consumption was not a traditional part of Māori society and was brought to Aotearoa by early Pākehā explorers and traders. The gendered structure of Victorian settler society differed from that of Māori society, and social sanctions against women smoking were not as prevalent in Māori society during the first century of Pākehā occupation in Aotearoa. Consequently, Māori and non-Māori female populations have different historical smoking trends, and these influence smoking patterns of today (Reid & Pouwhare 1991). In the 1950s there were small (if any) socio-economic differences in smoking patterns (Shaw *et al.* 1999). Similar proportions of Māori and non-Māori men and Māori women were smokers during this period, although non-Māori women had lower rates (Reid & Pouwhare 1991). Socio-economic differences emerged in the 1960s, and became increasingly marked during the 1980s and 1990s. Although smoking patterns did not always mirror social health differentials (Shaw *et al.* 1999), increased socio-economic gradients in smoking over the past three decades are now contributing to increasing inequalities in mortality.

Indeed social status has become clearly discernible in smoking patterns – smoking is more prevalent in more deprived areas (Salmond & Crampton 2000; Crampton *et al.* 2000), among the unemployed (Wilson 2000b), among workers in 'disadvantaged' occupational classes (Wilson 2000a), in low income households (O'Dea & Howden-Chapman 2000), and in crowded households (Howden-Chapman & Wilson 2000). Pākehā are advantaged in distributions of paid work, occupations, income, and area deprivation, which contributes substantially to their lower overall smoking rate (just over 20 per cent of the population aged 15 years and over) compared to that of Māori (over 40 per cent) (Ministry of Health 2001). Because smoking prevalence peaks in the young adult years, the younger age structure of the Māori population also accounts for some of the difference (Ministry of Health 2001).

Occupational segregation also impacts on health through differential exposures to environmental tobacco smoke. Six years after the Smokefree Environments Act 1990 came into force, workplace smoking restrictions were found to be effective for office but not for non-office workplaces: 28 per cent of Māori workers were exposed to second-hand smoke during working hours compared to only 19 per cent of the total workforce (National Research Bureau (NRB) 1996). This has flow-on effects for smoking uptake and smoking cessation.

A study of 1996 Census data on smoking by ethnicity, age, and area deprivation found that quit-rates were higher among Pākehā than among Māori (Crampton *et al.* 2000). Compared with Pākehā men, fewer Māori men became ex-smokers as age increased, and this was most pronounced among Māori men in the most deprived areas. Also pronounced was a decrease in the proportion of middle-aged Māori women ex-smokers with increasing deprivation. The least deprived areas included 60 per cent more ex-smokers than the most deprived areas. Giving up smoking or 'remaining quit' appears to be more difficult for people living in more deprived areas.

Recent tobacco control policies have reduced overall smoking prevalence 'but have had the paradoxical effect of increasing health inequalities' (Jarvis & Wardle 1999: 252). Although there was a larger absolute decrease in smoking prevalence among Māori between 1981 and 1996, the relative inequality increased. Māori smoking rates declined by 17 per cent (from 56 per cent to 46 per cent) while non-Māori rates declined by 26 per cent (from 32 per cent to 24 per cent) (Laugesen & Clements 1998). Further efforts to reduce smoking prevalence, unless they are concentrated on Māori, may only serve to further widen inequalities in death rates from smoking.

Based on 1996 smoking prevalence rates, and an excise tax level of $6 per packet of 20 cigarettes, the Crown receives at least $200 million each year in tobacco excise tax from Māori smokers alone (excluding GST).[3] Between 1992 and 1999, the total value of Treaty of Waitangi settlements amounted to a little over $635 million – just three years' worth of tobacco excise tax paid by Māori smokers. The total value of the Ngāi Tahu settlement amounted to $30 million, less than one year's tobacco tax contributed by Māori, as did the Tainui settlement and the 1992 Fisheries Settlement (each approximately $170 million) (Te Puni Kōkiri 2000). To take over $200 million a year from the population with the lowest incomes, highest unemployment rates, lowest levels of wealth and assets, the lowest economic living standards, and the highest prevalence of persistent smoking seems punitive and contradictory if the aim of increased tobacco tax is to decrease smoking prevalence.

Smoking remains a major contributor to health disparities and it is not uncommon for smoking behaviour to be attributed to individual choice. But this behaviour is strongly shaped by income, deprivation, occupation, and other factors that can be called intermediary factors (see Hill, Chapter 3). These intermediary factors are themselves the outcome of structural factors such as the continuing impacts of colonialism as well as gender and ethnicity. In addition, smoking has a greater economic impact on the Māori population, with tobacco tax constituting over half of that impact, compounding the effect of the underlying structural determinants.

This example of tobacco consumption and tobacco control shows how Māori uptake and duration of tobacco use is a result of colonial history and socially-determined segregation, how Māori pay a disproportionate amount of money to the government as a result, and how government policy can increase health disparities between Māori and non-Māori.

## Child poverty and the forces of racism

Poverty is not fixed – 'it is a structural problem to do with the unequal distribution of resources and opportunities' (UNICEF 2000 cited in D'Souza & Wood 2003). In New Zealand, child poverty is structured along ethnic lines. A Pākehā child is less than half as likely as a Māori child or Pacific child to be living in poverty.[4]

Around six out of ten children under 15 years of age in New Zealand are Pākehā, one in four is Māori, and one in ten is Pacific. Despite being a numerical majority, however, Pākehā children constitute a minority of children living in poverty.

The forces of racism discussed above structure poverty differentially for Māori and Pākehā children. This also means the impact of poverty on health is of a different magnitude for Pākehā children than for Māori (and Pacific) children. Between 1996 and 1999, the total number of Pākehā infants who died from Sudden Infant Death Syndrome (SIDS) was lower than the total number of Māori infants. The rate of SIDS among Māori in the most deprived areas (decile 10) was six times the rate of Pākehā infants in the most deprived areas (Te Rōpū Rangahau Hauora a Eru Pōmare, unpub.). Of children under 15 years of age affected by rheumatic fever, tuberculosis, or bronchiectasis (D'Souza & Wood 2003), or dying from injuries (Ajwani et al. 2003), Pākehā children were by far a minority.

In Aotearoa 'diseases of poverty' could equally well be termed 'diseases of colonisation and racism'. Therefore, to be truly effective, policies designed to reduce child poverty and alleviate its impact must take careful cognisance of the different lived realities of Pākehā children living in poverty compared to Māori and other non-Pākehā children living in poverty. Pākehā children living in poverty will have higher economic living standards (Krishnan et al. 2002).[5] Their length of exposure to poverty is likely to be shorter (Horsfield & Evans 1988).[6] Their families will own more material wealth and assets (Krishnan et al. 2002) and their grandparents will be financially better off (Cunningham et al. 2002). Their families will have more choice of housing because landlords, letting agents, real estate agents and mortgage lenders will feel more comfortable interacting with them and will believe their families to be more reliable, trustworthy tenants or mortgagees (Macdonald 1986; Māori Women's Housing Research Project 1991). They will not be subject to the same level of scrutiny by the police as their Māori counterparts, and if they are, the consequences will be less serious. Even if they offend at the same frequency, they will have far less contact with the police,[7] will experience fewer arrests, and will receive fewer convictions[8] (Fergusson et al. 2003a; 2003b).

Their school teachers will feel more confident interacting with them as students and communicating with their families about their progress, and less confident about doing these things with Māori students (Te Puni Kōkiri 2001). The vision of their future held by school management, governance, and teaching staff will be one of greater potential than that held for the Māori students (Te Puni Kōkiri 2001). This vision will affect decisions about the class the students are placed in, the seniority and qualifications of the teachers assigned to that class, the subjects the students are encouraged to take, and the careers counselling they are given (Jeffries 1998).

The nurse or doctor they are more likely to see if they become sick will feel more comfortable interacting with them and their parent or caregiver than they will with the Māori child and their family (McCreanor & Nairn 2002). This will affect the amount and type of information provided to them, the type of treatment provided and ongoing referrals (van Ryn & Burke 2000).

If their parents are beneficiaries, Pākehā children are more likely to receive a disability allowance for chronic conditions, and at a higher amount than that received by Māori or Pacific children (Howell & Hackwell 2003). Their illness will therefore have less impact on their family's financial position, and they will be more able to obtain needed health care and disability support.

While Pākehā children in poverty undoubtedly face significant economic barriers to good health and recovery, the non-financial barriers impacting on Māori children are both significant and comprehensive. Policies based on the experience of 'New Zealand' children living in poverty will undoubtedly help alleviate poverty for Māori children. However, they may not address the non-financial aspects that contribute to the extreme disparities in diseases of poverty among New Zealand children. Any strategies to address child poverty and its effects cannot ignore the way racism – in all its structural, institutional, and interpersonal forms – distributes privilege and penalty so that poverty produces differential health and social outcomes for children according to their ethnicity. Making New Zealand fit for all children requires all of us to steadfastly and courageously face up to the existence of racism in our society, the unequal distribution of resources and opportunities it produces, and the differential impact it has on the health of all our children.

## Conclusion

Differences in health outcomes between Māori and non-Māori are profound, deep-rooted and enduring. This chapter has illustrated these disparities by drawing on evidence from social epidemiology, and then providing a few examples that offer insights into how the disparities have come about and how they are maintained. The focus of this chapter has been to link health disparities to economic determinants, but in so doing it is clear that we cannot talk about economics alone when we want to consider how to redress the situation and move towards a more just and equitable society. The current economic situation for Māori and non-Māori is profoundly linked to the history of colonialism in Aotearoa and to embedded racism.

The interdependence of the education system, the labour market, and the welfare state means that New Zealand's tax and transfer policies, and the way they are implemented, require careful evaluation of their effect on Māori economic status and the flow-on health impacts. Significant widening of gaps between Māori and non-Māori in education, employment, income, and housing since the economic restructuring in the 1980s and 1990s signals a failure of the welfare state. The Crown and New Zealand society must act to address discriminatory policy and practice across all arenas if the right to good health for all is to be achieved. The vigour of Māori development must be supported by intensified efforts to dismantle structural barriers, only some of which have been discussed in this chapter.

# 3. Socio-economic inequalities in health

## Sarah Hill

Health, like most resources, is distributed unevenly throughout society. In the discipline of social epidemiology, the focus is not on individual differences in health, but on measuring and comparing the average health of different population groups, defining these by gender, ethnicity, geography, occupation, and many other social parameters.

When the health of different population groups is compared, common patterns start to emerge. Those groups that enjoy the most advantaged positions in society – good educational achievement, secure jobs, adequate income, comfortable housing – are also those that enjoy the best health. And those whose position in society is more marginal – those with few qualifications, insecure or erratic employment, low income and poor quality housing – have the most fragile health.

Inequalities in the distribution of health have been described in many different societies, including Aotearoa New Zealand (Marmot *et al.* 1978; Black *et al.* 1980; Rose 1981; Wilkinson 1996; Pamuk *et al.* 1998; Berkman & Kawachi 2000; Davey Smith *et al.* 2002; Mackenbach & Bakker 2002; National Health Committee 1998; Ministry of Health 2000). The influence of social factors on health is enormous: in Aotearoa, people in the most advantaged tenth of society have a life expectancy eight years longer than those in the most disadvantaged tenth (Salmond & Crampton 2000). By contrast, few medical interventions can boast such a profound effect on survival.

This chapter sets out the epidemiological evidence for health inequalities in the New Zealand population, concentrating on the distribution of health by socio-economic position. Much of this evidence has emerged over the past 10 years, which have seen an increased focus on understanding and reducing social inequalities in health (National Health Committee 1998; Ministry of Health 2000; Pearce & Ellison-Loschmann 2002; King 2000; Ministry of Health 2002). Shifting trends in health disparities remind us that these patterns are not fixed: contemporary social, economic, and health environments will shape the way health is distributed in the New Zealand society of the future.

# Framing inequalities in health

## What causes health inequalities?

Why are some groups of people healthier than others? Differences in lifestyle factors such as smoking and diet, different use of health services, and specific environmental hazards are some of the explanations offered for variations in the health of population groups (Pearce *et al*. 1983b; Marmot 1999; Macintyre 1997).

While all these factors probably contribute to health inequalities, in themselves they provide only part of the explanation. A more fundamental question is why are some population groups more likely than others to experience harmful lifestyle, health care, and environmental characteristics (or, to put it another way, why do other groups experience favourable characteristics?). The real drivers of health inequalities lie deeper than these intermediary factors – in the way society distributes those resources that are the basic prerequisites of good health (including material wealth, housing, education, and job security).

## A framework for examining health inequalities

In New Zealand, the Ministry of Health has developed an 'intervention framework to improve health and reduce inequalities' (National Health Committee 1998; Ministry of Health 2002), a version of which is shown below (Figure 3.1). This framework illustrates the way in which health inequalities reflect the unequal distribution of those resources that are the basic foundations for good health (*structural determinants*). Inequalities in these underlying factors are then played out along various pathways (intermediary pathways) – including biological, behavioural, and environmental experiences – and in interactions with *health services*. The framework includes a fourth element in which health outcomes themselves have a 'feedback' effect or *impact* on the underlying social and economic determinants of health.

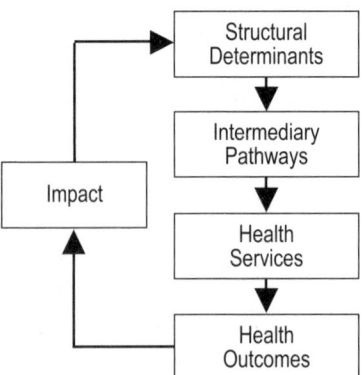

*Figure 3.1: A framework of inequalities in health. (Adapted from National Health Committee 1998 and Ministry of Health 2002)*

This framework is a very simplified representation of the complex and interconnected processes underpinning health and disease; nevertheless, it provides a useful model for examining inequalities in health. We will start by looking at health outcomes themselves, considering how life expectancy, risk of death, and the occurrence of disease vary across different population groups. We will then look behind these health outcomes at those pathway factors that contribute to health inequalities. These factors include disparities in health services provision, unequal exposure to risk factors for disease and injury, and the unequal distribution of socio-economic resources in Aotearoa.

## Markers and pathways of inequality

Since the focus here is on the relationship between socio-economic position and health, some way of measuring people's socio-economic resources is needed. Income, education, occupation, housing status, and car access have all been used as measures or markers of socio-economic position (Ministry of Health 2002; Roberts *et al.* 1996). Some of these measures (such as income or car access) relate to tangible material resources, while others (such as occupational class) are more a marker of a person's place in the social hierarchy.

Commentators have debated which of these dimensions play more important roles in mediating health outcome. Some focus on material pathways to health and disease, highlighting the ways in which poverty limits access to basic physical resources such as adequate housing and nutrition (Davey Smith *et al.* 1994). Others place more emphasis on a person's status in society and the relationship between that status and their state of health, including the psycho-social stresses experienced by those with lower social status and how these stresses are played out in biological terms (Wilkinson 1996, 1999).

It seems likely that both material and psycho-social mechanisms play a part in the development of health inequalities. In practice, most researchers use whatever measures are available to them at the time. None of these measures fully captures the complexity of a person's place in society, including the resources, opportunities, and social support available to them. Nevertheless by using a variety of measures we can build up a picture of the way in which health relates to a person's socio-economic situation. However this relationship is measured, the spectrum of socio-economic position is itself a consequence of those basic societal forces that drive the unequal distribution of the goods of society, including material, political, and social resources (of which health is one) (Williams 1997).

## Socio-economic position and ethnicity

In Aotearoa – as in many countries – socio-economic position is often closely aligned with ethnicity. The experience of colonisation means Māori are underrepresented in those groups with the greatest share of economic resources (Reid *et al.* 2000; Robson 2004; Ministry of Social Development 2005). Pacific and other recent migrant groups also experience a degree of marginalisation and tend to have fewer socio-economic resources (Ministry of Social Development 2005).

While recognising the relationship between ethnicity and socio-economic position, it is important to distinguish between these two factors when looking at health inequalities. Poorer socio-economic position drives some of the difference in health between ethnic groups, but there are other important explanations at work – such as colonisation and racism (Reid *et al.* 2000; Robson 2004; Harris *et al.* 2006). Furthermore, socio-economic disparities exist within as well as between ethnic groups, just as ethnic health disparities persist within the same socio-economic grouping (Pearce *et al.*1993; Sporle *et al* 2002; Reid *et al.* 2000; Fawcett *et al.* 2006). The relationship between ethnicity, socio-economic position and health is also explored in Chapter 2 (Robson) and Chapter 4 (Cunningham) of this book.

## What patterns of health inequality do we see in Aotearoa New Zealand?

*Inequalities in life expectancy and the risk of death*

The most stark level at which health inequalities are seen is in the risk of death. The fact that, compared to others, some population groups have a higher death rate in younger age groups provides a crude but powerful measure of these groups' different health experiences. A person's risk of death may be represented as life expectancy (the length of time an average person would live if they experienced contemporary conditions throughout their life), or mortality rate (the statistical risk of death a person is subject to at a particular point in time).[1]

*Inequalities by occupational class*

Neil Pearce produced some of the earliest work on social inequalities in health in New Zealand (Pearce *et al.* 1983a, 1983b). Pearce and colleagues took death records from 1975 to 1977 and compared these with population counts from the 1976 Census, using these two sets of information to calculate mortality rates (or risk of death) in men aged 15 to 64 years (Pearce *et al.* 1983a). They grouped the men according to their stated occupation, based on a system known as the Elley-Irving index. This index produces six grades of occupational or 'social' class, ranging from one (including doctors, lawyers, and other 'professionals') to six (including cleaners, freight handlers, and unskilled labourers) (Elley & Irving 1972, 1976). Pearce found a clear gradient in overall mortality, with men in higher occupational classes experiencing low risk of death compared with those in lower occupational classes (Figure 3.2).

This occupational gradient in mortality was seen across all causes of death (Pearce *et al.* 1983b), and was most noticeable for deaths due to accidents, lung disease, diabetes and related conditions, and mental disorders. Inequalities in death risk were less pronounced for heart disease and cancer, although a strong gradient was evident for some specific cancers such as lung and liver (Pearce

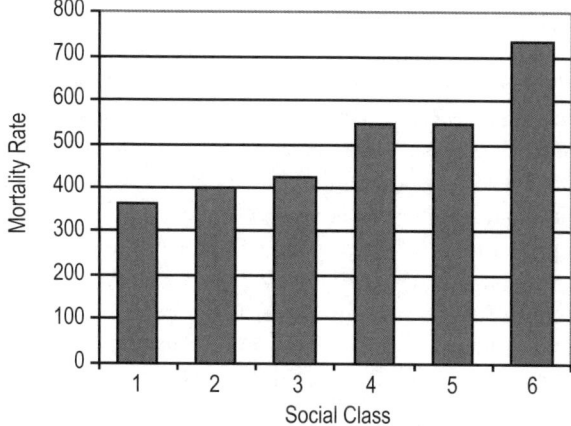

*Figure 3.2: Mortality rates (per 100,000 per year) in 15–64 year old New Zealand men by Elley-Irving index, 1975–7. Mortality rates are age-standardised to Segi's world population. (Data from Pearce et al. 1983a)*

& Howard 1986).

Over time, Pearce and colleagues expanded this work to look at both social and ethnic differences in mortality rates among New Zealand men (Pearce *et al.* 2002; Sporle *et al.* 2002). They found that occupational class and ethnicity were each independently related to risk of death: within the same occupational group there were clear mortality differences between Māori and non-Māori men, while a social class gradient was apparent amongst both Māori and non-Māori men.

Pearce's work shows the risk of premature death in the New Zealand population is related to occupational class. Men in unskilled jobs, working as labourers, freight handlers and cleaners, for example, have a higher risk of early death compared with men in professional and managerial jobs, such as those working as doctors and lawyers.

## Inequalities by small area deprivation (NZDep)

The development of the New Zealand Deprivation Index (NZDep) in the 1990s provided an enormously valuable tool for studying inequalities in health in Aotearoa. NZDep is a scale of material deprivation, based on the aggregated characteristics of individuals living in the same geographical area (Crampton *et al.* 1997a; Salmond *et al.* 1998). An NZDep score can thus be thought of as reflecting the average socio-economic experience of people living in a particular area, captured through measures of income, transport, living space, home ownership, employment, qualifications, and support. Unlike the Elley-Irving index (used by Pearce and colleagues), the application of NZDep in research doesn't require collection of individual information on occupation or other aspects of socio-economic position. This makes it much easier to use NZDep for groups who may not be in the paid workforce (especially women, children, and older people). An NZDep score can be obtained on the basis of an individual's home address, so it is easy to use with routine data sources such as hospitalisation and other health care records.

The application of NZDep scores to death records shows how the risk of premature death varies by socio-economic position for the whole New Zealand population. What we find is a continuous gradient in mortality, with the lowest risk of death in the least deprived areas (NZDep decile 1) and the highest risk in the most deprived areas (NZDep decile 10) (Figure 3.3). The same pattern is seen for men and women, across ethnic groups (Māori, Pacific and other), and across age groups (Salmond & Crampton 2000). These findings demonstrate the fundamental influence of socio-economic circumstances for the health of all groups in Aotearoa.

These mortality rates can be used to calculate life expectancy by deprivation decile. Life expectancy shows the reverse pattern to mortality: those living in the most advantaged areas enjoy the highest life expectancy, while those living in the most disadvantaged areas have the lowest life expectancy (Figure 3.4). The difference in life expectancy at birth between the least and most deprived tenths of New Zealand society is approximately nine years in males, and seven years in females.

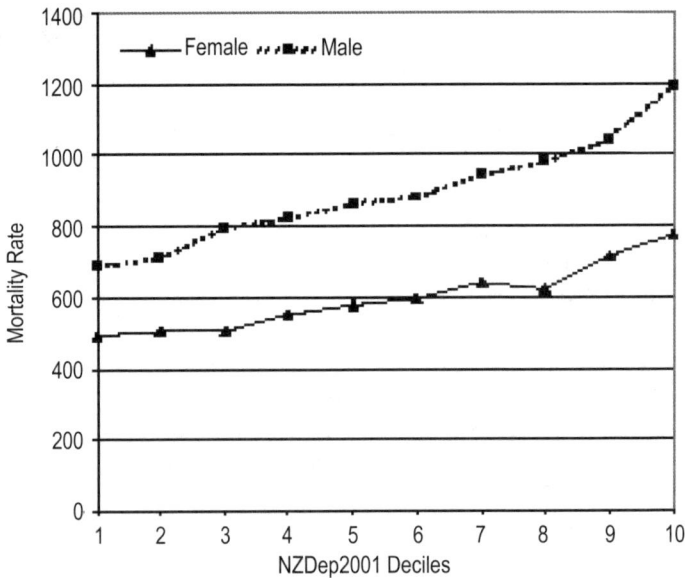

*Figure 3.3: Mortality rates (per 100,000 per year) by deprivation of area of residence (NZDep2001 decile), total New Zealand population, 2000–2. Mortality rates are age-standardised to the 2001 Census population. NZDep2001 deciles: 1=least deprived, 10=most deprived. (Data from Statistics New Zealand, 2006)*

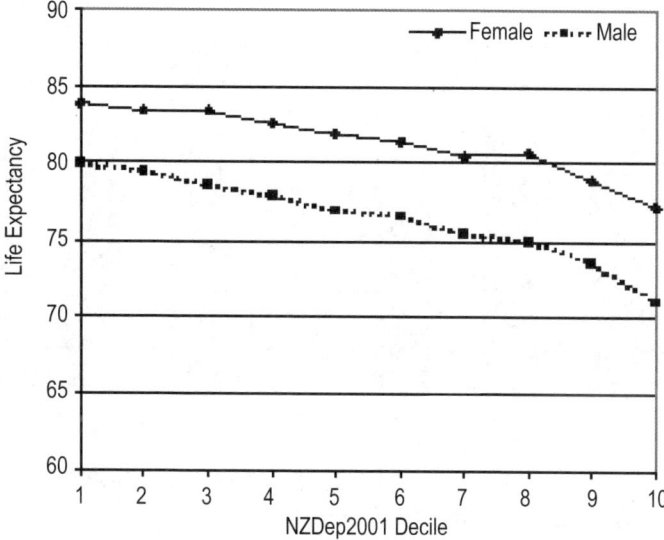

*Figure 3.4: Life expectancy (years) by deprivation of area of residence (NZDep2001 decile), total New Zealand population, 2000–2. NZDep2001 deciles: 1=least deprived, 10=most deprived. (Data from Statistics New Zealand 2006)*

## The New Zealand Census Mortality Study

The development of the New Zealand Census Mortality Study (NZCMS) was a major milestone in describing and understanding health inequalities in Aotearoa. The NZCMS uses linked census and mortality records from the whole New Zealand population to track mortality risk by ethnicity and socio-economic position, providing time-series data from 1981 onwards (Blakely 2002a; Blakely *et al.* 2005; Ajwani *et al.* 2003; Fawcett *et al.* 2006). This database overcomes many of the shortcomings inherent in previous studies. Since socio-economic position is measured *prior* to mortality there is less risk of reverse causality (that is, we can be confident that poorer socio-economic position preceded a deterioration in health, rather than the other way around). Furthermore, we can look at patterns in mortality for the whole population (including women[2]) by several different individual or household measures of socio-economic position – such as income, education, and occupation – using the same measures over time to get accurate time-series data. Finally, the NZCMS provided New Zealand's first accurate picture of ethnic differences in mortality by applying the same self-identified ethnic categories to both population and death counts (Ajwani *et al.* 2003; Blakely *et al.* 2002b). The NZCMS shows a clear gradient in mortality by categories of income, education, and occupation, with highest mortality in the most disadvantaged and lowest mortality in the most advantaged groups (Blakely *et al.* 2005) (Figures 3.5 and 3.6).

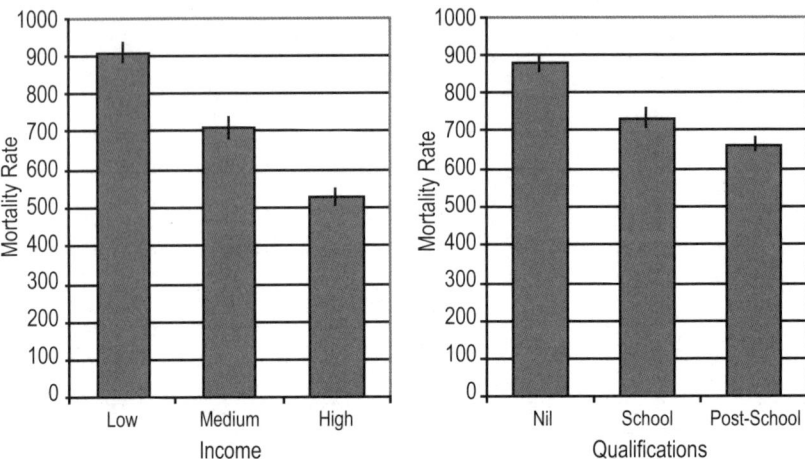

*Figure 3.5: Mortality rates (per 100,000/year) in 25–77 year old New Zealand men by income and education (qualifications), 1996–9. Mortality rates are age- and ethnicity-standardised to the 1991 Census population. Income refers to annual household income in 1996 NZ$, equivalised for household size using the Jensen equivalisation index (see Blakely 2002a). Income categories are low (<$26,109), medium ($26,110–$43,015) and high (>$43,015). Vertical lines represent 95% confidence intervals. (Data from Blakely et al. 2005)*

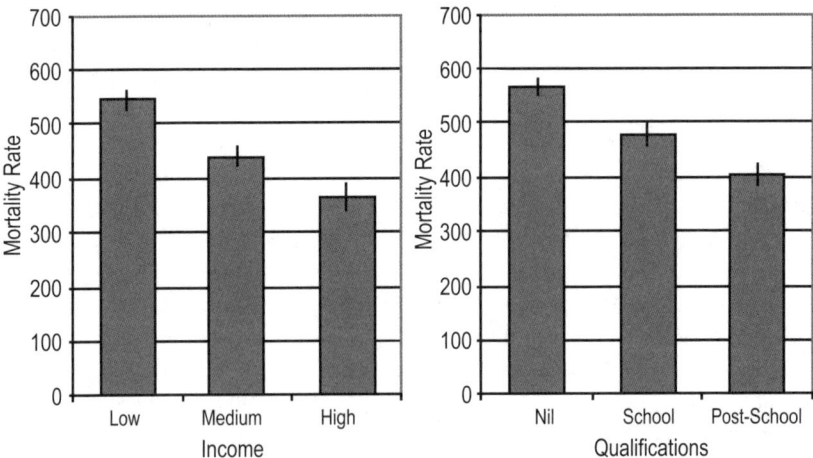

*Figure 3.6: Mortality rates (per 100,000/year) in 25–77 year old New Zealand women by income and education (qualifications), 1996–9. Mortality rates are age- and ethnicity-standardised to the 1991 Census population. Income refers to annual household income in 1996 NZ$, equivalised for household size using the Jensen equivalisation index (see Blakely 2002a). Income categories are low (<$26,109), medium ($26,110–$43,015) and high (>$43,015). Vertical lines represent 95% confidence intervals. (Data from Blakely et al. 2005)*

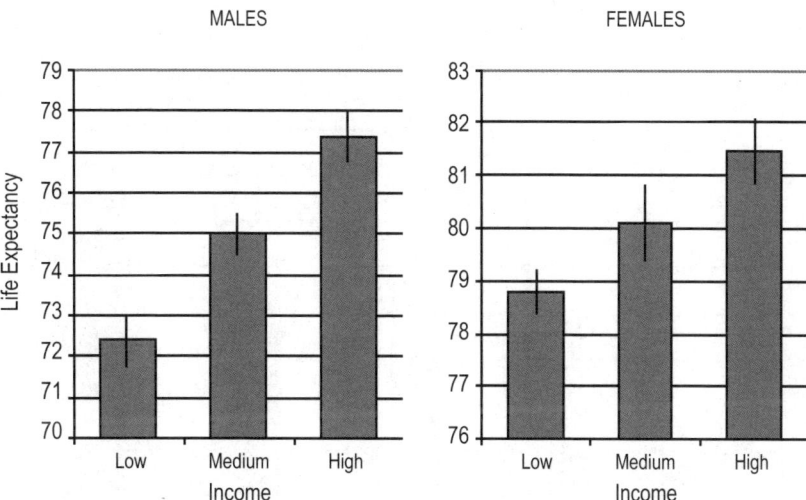

*Figure 3.7: Life expectancy at birth (years) for men and women by income, 1996–9. Income refers to annual household income in 1996 NZ$, equivalised for household size using the Jensen equivalisation index (see Blakely 2002a). Income categories are low (<$26,109), medium ($26,110–$43,015) and high (>$43,015). Vertical lines represent 95% confidence intervals. (Data from Blakely et al. 2005)*

Mortality rates by income have been used to calculate life expectancy at birth for different income groups. In the 1996–9 period, all-cause mortality was 70 per cent higher in men and 50 per cent higher in women, comparing the lowest third with the highest third of the population (by income). Translated into life expectancy, this represents a gap of 5.0 years in men and 2.7 years in women (Figure 3.7).

At a disease-specific level, inequalities in mortality risk are evident across a wide range of conditions including heart disease, cancer, lung disease, injury, and suicide (Blakely *et al.* 2005; Shaw *et al.* 2005b; Shaw *et al.* 2006).

In summary, the New Zealand Census Mortality Study shows that the risk of early death is highest in those people with low incomes and fewer formal qualifications. In Aotearoa, people with high incomes and post-school qualifications are least likely to die early.

Other New Zealand studies have also demonstrated social gradients in mortality from heart disease (Riddell 2005; Kawachi *et al.* 1991), stroke (Kawachi *et al.* 1991), and cancer (Pearce & Bethwaite 1997). Several researchers have found that socio-economic differences in mortality are more pronounced for those conditions thought to be amenable to appropriate health care (Sporle *et al.* 2002; Ministry of Health 2004b; Marshall *et al.* 1993). This pattern suggests that disadvantaged groups in society are unable to access adequate levels of health care, further contributing to their poor health status.

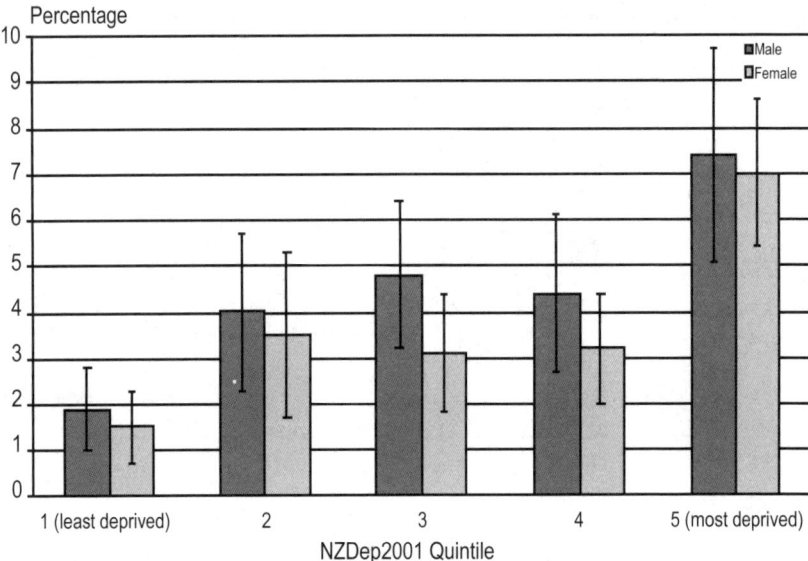

*Figure 3.8: Prevalence of diagnosed diabetes in New Zealand adults by area of deprivation (NZDep2001 quintile), 2002/3. Prevalence is age-standardised to the 2001 Census population. Vertical lines represent 95% confidence intervals. (Data from Ministry of Health 2004a)*

### Inequalities in disease and ill-health

Health inequalities exist across a wide range of diseases and conditions. New Zealanders with poorer socio-economic positions have higher rates of asthma, diabetes (Figure 3.8), heart disease, lung cancer, cervical cancer, musculoskeletal disorders, injury, infectious diseases, mental disorders, and complications associated with pregnancy (Salmond *et al.* 1998; Salmond *et al.* 1999; Riddell 2005; McFadden *et al.* 2004; Taylor *et al.* 2004; Salmond & Crampton 2000; Ministry of Health 2004a; Whitlock *et al.* 2003).

Work by Davis and colleagues shows that, compared to others, people in lower occupational classes (measured by the Elley-Irving index) spend a greater proportion of their lives suffering from ill-health or disability (Davis *et al.* 1999). Thus people in more disadvantaged circumstances not only have shorter life expectancy, but also spend more of their lives living with the effects of disease or injury.

### Inequalities in child health

Inequalities in health are apparent for children as well as adults. Studies of disease and death risk in New Zealand children show that socio-economic position influences health from a very early age through to adulthood, regardless of a change in socio-economic circumstances.

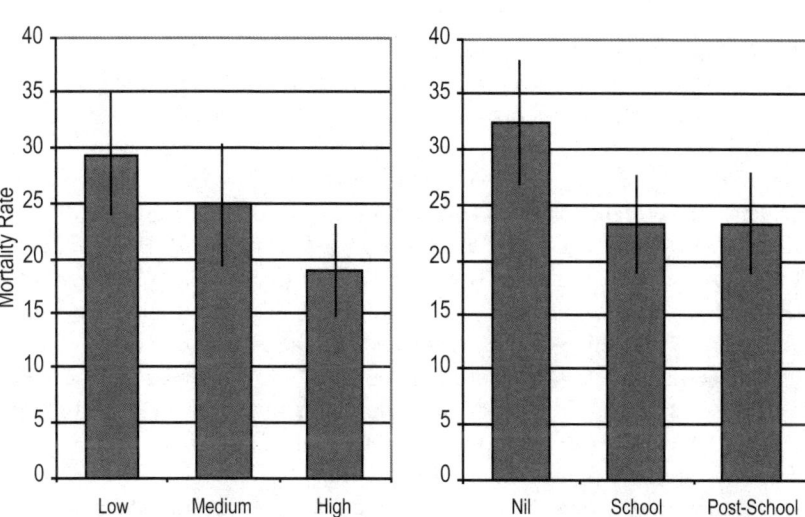

*Figure 3.9: Mortality rates (per 100,000 per year) in New Zealand children aged 1–14 by household income and maternal education (qualifications), 1996–9. Mortality rates are age-standardised to the 1991 Census population. Income refers to annual household income in 1996 NZ$, equivalised for household size using the Jensen equivalisation index (see Blakely 2002a). Income categories are low (<$20,600), medium ($20,601–$33,000) and high (>$33,000). Vertical lines represent 95% confidence intervals. Data from Shaw et al. 2005a.*

Using data from the NZCMS, Shaw and colleagues examined the risk of death in children according to the socio-economic characteristics of the adults with whom they lived (Shaw *et al*. 2005a). They found a consistent gradient in mortality for children aged 1 to 14 years, with greater risk of death among children living in disadvantaged households (Figure 3.9). This pattern was evident across a broad range of conditions including road traffic accidents and other injuries, communicable diseases, asthma, and lung infections (Shaw *et al*. 2005c).

Children's experience of socio-economic disadvantage was also linked with health status in the Dunedin longitudinal study[3] (Silva & Stanton 1996). Investigators found that children born into less advantaged families (measured by parents' occupational groupings) were more likely to have compromised health at birth (Poulton *et al*. 2002). The socio-economic conditions in which children grew up were also related to several measures of health status in adulthood, including cardiovascular health, dental health, and substance abuse. Furthermore, the effect of socio-economic disadvantage in childhood persisted even when children moved into higher socio-economic groups as they grew older (Poulton *et al*. 2002).

## Inequalities in health services

Despite having higher rates of hospital admissions, people living in more deprived circumstances seem to face greater barriers to health service use, and are unable to access a level of medical care appropriate to their needs. Several New Zealand studies have found that people with fewer socio-economic resources have higher rates of conditions thought to be preventable through adequate health care (Pearce *et al.* 1991, 1993; Marshall *et al.* 1993; Salmond & Crampton 2000; Jackson & Tobias 2001; Ministry of Health 2004b, 2005). People living in more deprived areas are less likely to be able to see their family doctor when they need to (Ministry of Health 2004a).

Marshall and colleagues looked at amenable and non-amenable mortality in New Zealand men aged 15–64 years during the mid-1980s (Marshall *et al.* 1993). ('Amenable mortality' refers to those deaths that could be expected to be prevented by the provision of appropriate health services.) When they compared mortality rates by occupational class, they found gradients in both amenable and non-amenable mortality. The gradient in amenable mortality was even more pronounced than that for non-amenable mortality: men in the lowest occupational group had an amenable mortality rate more than three times higher than men in the highest occupational group, while the difference for non-amenable mortality was two-fold (Marshall *et al.* 1993).

Similar approaches have been used to examine socio-economic differences in avoidable hospitalisations – that is, hospitalisations that could have been avoided through preventive and primary health services (Salmond & Crampton 2000; Jackson & Tobias 2001). Work by Salmond and Crampton shows a gradient in both avoidable and non-avoidable hospitalisations across deciles of deprivation (Salmond & Crampton 2000). The Ministry of Health reports a similar gradient in ambulatory-sensitive hospitalisations – that is, hospitalisations that could be prevented through appropriate outpatient and primary health care (Ministry of Health 2005) (Figure 3.10).

Data from the New Zealand Health Survey 2002/3 confirm that people living in deprived areas experience greater difficulty in accessing primary health care (Ministry of Health 2004a). Adults living in higher deprivation areas were less likely to take up screening opportunities, and were more likely to report having needed to see a doctor in the last 12 months and being unable to do so (Figure 3.11).

These findings suggest that New Zealanders with fewer socio-economic resources face barriers that prevent them from accessing an appropriate level of health care. This lack of adequate health care in turn contributes to socio-economic inequalities in health outcomes.

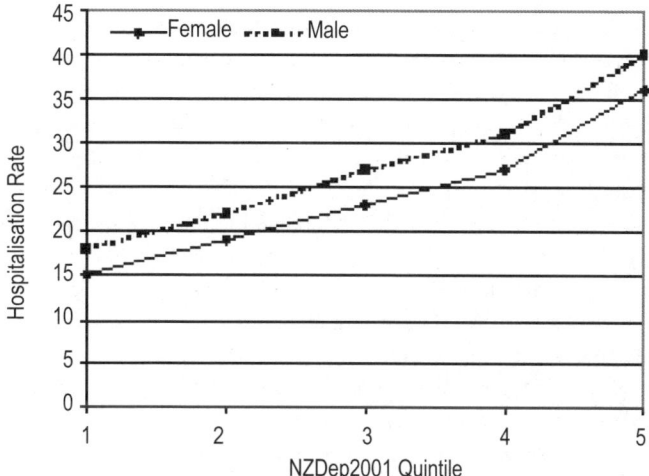

*Figure 3.10: Ambulatory-sensitive hospitalisations (per 1000 per year) by deprivation of area of residence (NZDep2001 quintile), total New Zealand population, 2001–4. NZDep2001 quintiles: 1=least deprived, 5=most deprived. Rates are age-standardised to the 2001 Census population. (Data from Ministry of Health 2005)*

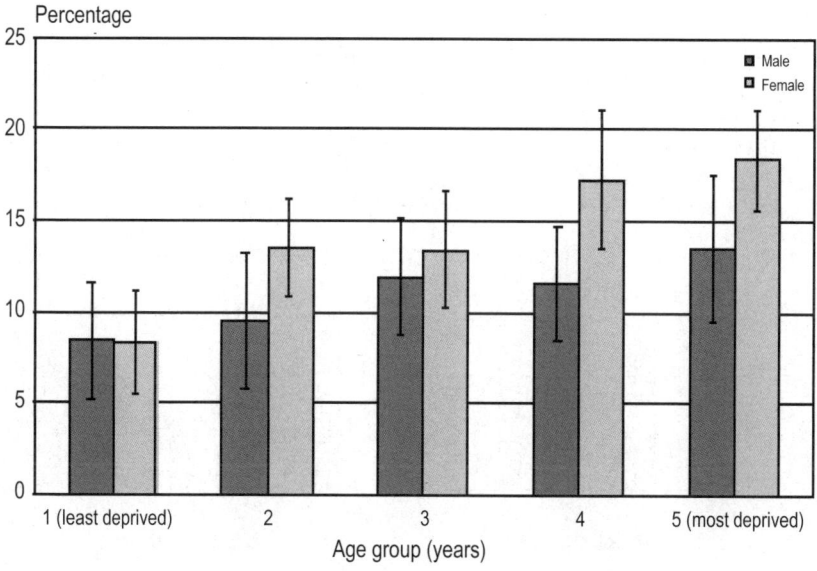

*Figure 3.11: Percentage of adults having unmet need for general practitioner in the last 12 months, by deprivation of area of residence (NZDep2001 quintile), 2002/3. Percentage rates are age-standardised to the 2001 Census population. Vertical lines represent 95% confidence intervals. (Data from Ministry of Health 2004a)*

*Inequalities in relation to intermediary pathways*

We have seen that there are inequalities in the distribution of health and disease in New Zealand society, and in health service use. Less advantaged population groups are more likely to be sick, less likely to receive health care appropriate to their needs, and more likely to die early compared with those in relatively advantaged groups.

Intermediary pathways to health outcomes include risk factors for disease and injury. These are distributed unevenly throughout the New Zealand population, with unhealthy characteristics more common in those with fewer socio-economic resources. These characteristics include smoking, obesity, high blood pressure, and poor diet.

There is a well-recognised association between socio-economic circumstances and tobacco use, with higher smoking rates in less advantaged population groups (Whitlock *et al.* 1997; Borman *et al.* 1999; Salmond & Crampton 2000; Crampton *et al.* 2000; Hill *et al.* 2003; Ministry of Health 2004a). Data from the 1996 Census showed that people with no formal qualifications had a smoking rate three times higher than that of people with tertiary qualifications (Borman *et al.* 1999). Smokers from less advantaged groups are also less likely to successfully quit smoking (Hill *et al.* 2003).

Data from the 2002/3 Health Survey show people living in more deprived areas are more likely have high blood pressure, less likely to be physically active and more likely to be obese (Ministry of Health 2004a) (Figure 3.12). They also tend to have a lower fruit and vegetable intake (Figure 3.13).

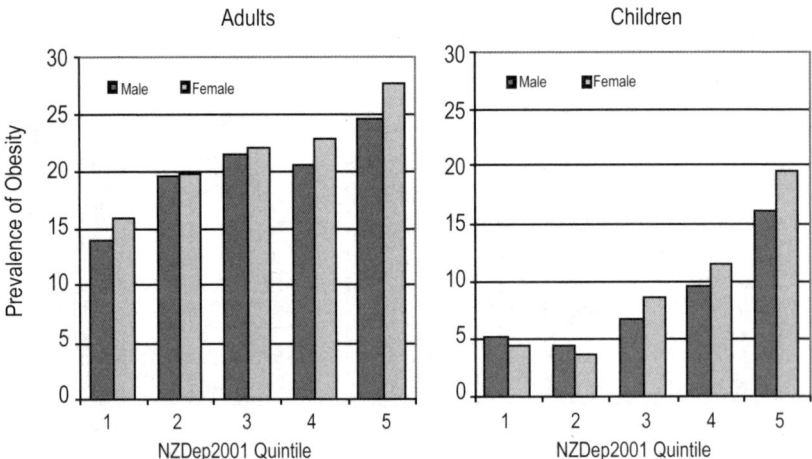

*Figure 3.12. Prevalence of obesity by deprivation of area of residence (NZDep2001 quintile), New Zealand adults (15 years and over) and children (5–14 years), 2003/04. NZDep2001 quintilequintiles: 1=least deprived, 5=most deprived. Prevalence in adults is age-standardised to the WHO world population (prevalence in children is not age-standardised). (Unpublished Data from Public Health Intelligence, Ministry of Health, 2006)*

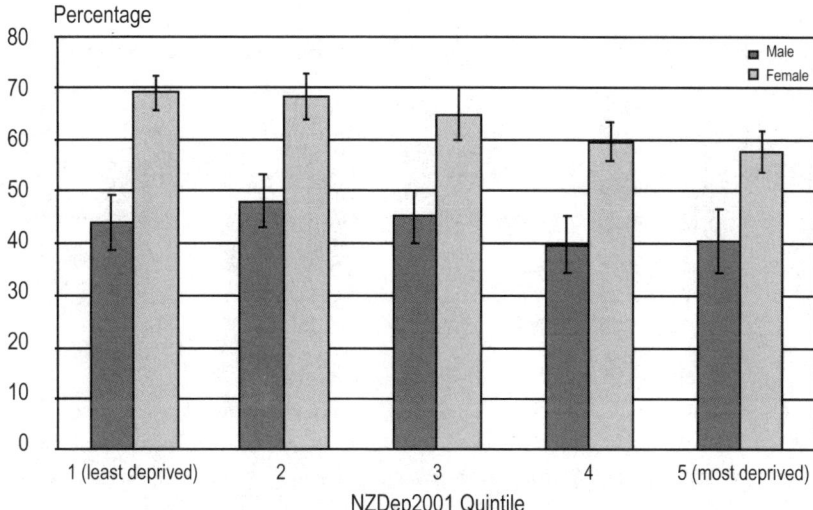

*Figure 3.13: Fruit intake (two or more servings per day) by deprivation of area of residence (NZDep2001 quintiles), New Zealand adults 2002/3. Prevalence is age-standardised to the 2001 Census population. Vertical lines represent 95% confidence intervals. (Data from Ministry of Health 2004a)*

New Zealand children also experience unequal exposure to risk factors for injury and disease. Babies are more likely to be born at low birthweight if their fathers belong to a lower occupational class (Borman *et al.* 1990). The Dunedin longitudinal study found that children from more advantaged families performed better on learning tests and exhibited fewer behavioural problems than those from disadvantaged households (Silva & Stanton 1996).

An Auckland study found that pedestrian injury risk (measured as the average number of streets crossed each day) was higher in children from less advantaged households (Figure 3.14) (Roberts *et al.* 1996). This unequal risk exposure correlates closely with higher rates of road traffic injury in children from poor households (Shaw *et al.* 2005b).

These findings illustrate how less advantaged groups in society face greater risk of disease and injury. The authors of this study comment that children's differential exposure to pedestrian injury risk 'underscores the unequal societal distribution of the health advantages and disadvantages of car travel. Children from families without a car receive none of the benefits of car travel but a greater share of the risks' (Roberts *et al.* 1996).

Public health interventions also tend to be unevenly distributed, and often have their greatest impact in those groups already at lower risk. A recent Auckland study found that 'walking school buses' (an intervention aimed at increasing children's physical activity while improving their safety) were most concentrated in areas of relative socio-economic advantage where children already have the lowest risk of pedestrian injury (Collins & Kearns 2005).

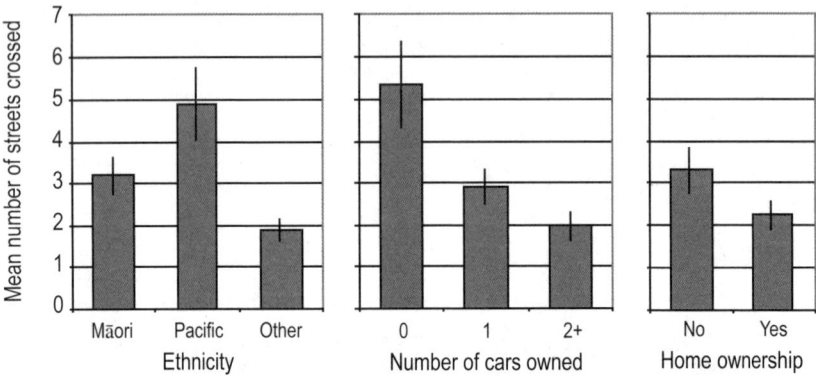

*Figure 3.14: Mean number of streets crossed each day by six- and nine-year-old Auckland schoolchildren, by ethnicity, number of cars owned and home ownership, 1994. Number of cars owned and home ownership refer to children's parents. Vertical lines represent 95% confidence intervals. (Data from Roberts et al. 1996)*

In summary, adults and children living in disadvantaged circumstances have greater exposure to risk factors for disease and injury. New Zealanders with more socio-economic resources are relatively protected from the causes of disease and ill-health.

## Inequalities in the determinants of health

In the final part of this section we examine inequalities in one of the underlying determinants of health, the distribution of socio-economic resources within New Zealand society.

Household income is an important marker of how socio-economic resources are distributed unevenly across the population.[4] In Aotearoa, the top 20 per cent of households have three times as much disposable income as the bottom 20 per cent (Ministry of Social Development 2005). Another way of measuring income distribution is the Gini coefficient: this ranges from 0 for populations with complete income equality (that is, everyone has the same income) to 100 for populations with complete inequality (that is, one person earns all the income there is).[5] New Zealand has a Gini coefficient of 33.9, indicating greater income inequality than the OECD average (median 30.1) (Figure 3.15) (Ministry of Social Development 2005).

Households that are more likely to have a low income include those with sole parents, three or more dependent children, adults belonging to ethnic groups other than Pākehā/New Zealand European, and those living in rented accommodation (Ministry of Social Development 2005).

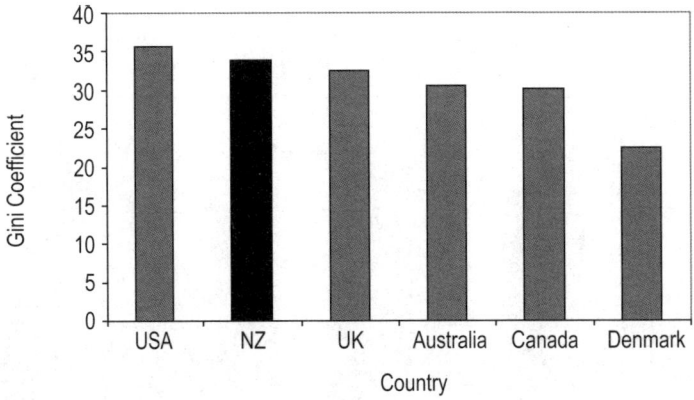

*Figure 3.15: Gini coefficient for New Zealand and other OECD countries, 2000. OECD median = 30.1. (Data from Ministry of Social Development 2005)*

## How have patterns of health inequality changed over time?

We have seen that health outcomes, access to health services, and the determinants of health are distributed unevenly throughout New Zealand society. But has this always been the case, or have these patterns changed over time?

The answer to both questions is probably 'Yes'. This section looks at trends in health outcomes and their socio-economic determinants.

### Trends in total mortality and life expectancy

The New Zealand Census Mortality Study provides excellent time-series data on mortality patterns from the early 1980s onwards. Figure 3.16 shows all-cause mortality by household income for men and women.

Two patterns are immediately evident from these graphs. First, mortality risk fell in all income groups over the 1980s and 1990s. Second, a strong income gradient persisted in both men and women throughout these two decades, with higher mortality in the lowest income group, and lower mortality in the highest income group.

A closer look shows that the slope or gradient of mortality risk across the three income groups remains approximately the same over the four time periods.[6] This slope represents the 'absolute' inequality in mortality risk.[7] At the same time, the size of the mortality risk has reduced in all three income groups. This means the difference in mortality risk between the highest and lowest income groups has increased in 'relative' terms.[8] A shorthand way of describing this pattern is to say that *absolute inequalities in mortality risk remained static* from the early 1980s to the late 1990s, while *relative inequalities in mortality risk increased*.

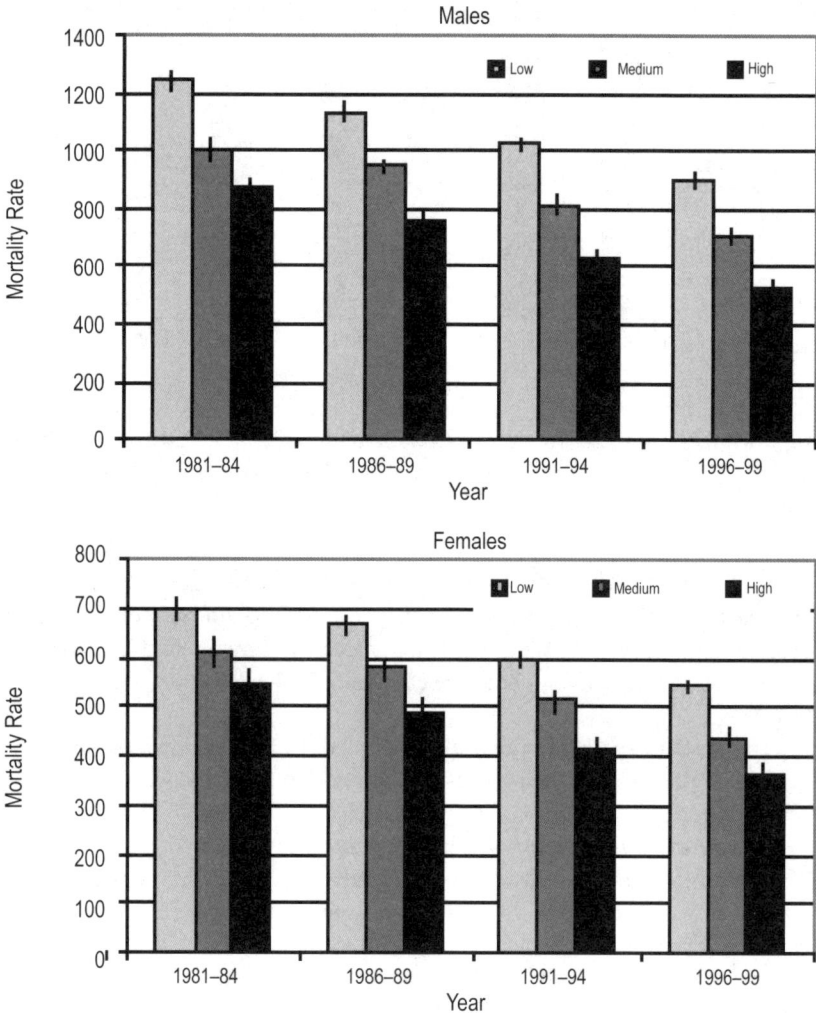

*Figure 3.16: Mortality rates (per 100,000 per year) in New Zealanders aged 25–77 by household income, 1981–99. Mortality rates are age- and ethnicity-standardised to the 1991 Census population. Vertical lines represent 95% confidence intervals. (Data from Blakely et al. 2005)*

Absolute and relative inequalities are two slightly different ways of thinking about the distribution of health or ill health in a population. Ideally, we want to see a reduction in both absolute and relative inequalities. However, in the context of a gradual decline in premature mortality (such as Aotearoa has experienced over the past 100 years), reducing or stable differences in absolute mortality, and stable or increasing gaps in relative mortality are often observed.[9] This pattern suggests that more privileged groups in society are the first to benefit from advances in standards of living and health care (Victora *et al.* 2000). If health gains were shared evenly by all population groups, a decline in both absolute and relative inequalities would be seen.

The patterns shown in Figure 3.16 are roughly similar to those described by Pearce and colleagues. In other words, the distribution of health in the New Zealand population became more unequal (in relative terms) between the 1980s and the 1990s. Several commentators have noted that this period coincides with an era of radical social and economic reform in New Zealand's public sector (Howden-Chapman & Tobias 2000; Sporle *et al.* 2002; Blakely *et al.* 2005). The implication is that these reforms were responsible for widening gaps in the health of New Zealanders.

Other research suggests that while mortality risk declined for all New Zealanders from the early 1980s onwards, people in worse socio-economic circumstances were more likely to be living with disability and disease. Davis and colleagues looked at changes in life expectancy from the early 1980s to the early 1990s (Davis *et al.* 1999). They found a modest increase in life expectancy across all social groups, reflecting the decline in mortality risk described above. When they adjusted for disability, however, they found that only higher social groups experienced an increase in healthy life expectancy (that is, healthy or disability-free years of life). In other social groups, increases in life expectancy were counterbalanced by an increase in years lived with disability.

## Trends in specific diseases

More variable time-trends are evident at the level of specific causes of death such as heart disease, cancer, and suicide. The distribution of heart disease by socio-economic status has changed markedly, coming almost full circle over the past 50 years. In the early 1960s heart disease appeared to be more common in New Zealand men from higher occupational classes (Copplestone & Rose 1967). By the mid-1970s this pattern had reversed, with the highest rates of heart disease in the lowest occupational classes (Pearce *et al.* 1983b). This social gradient in heart disease became even more pronounced during the 1980s (Kawachi *et al.* 1991); however, more recent data suggest that since the 1990s it has started to decline again (Blakely *et al.* 2005).

Changing socio-economic gradients are also evident in the risk of cancer and suicide. Inequalities in cancer mortality appeared to increase from the 1980s to the 1990s, with particularly pronounced increases for lung, breast and colorectal cancer (Blakely *et al.* 2005; Shaw *et al.* 2005b; Shaw *et al.* 2006). Suicide likewise changed from a relatively equal profile in the early 1980s to a much more marked social gradient in the late 1990s, particularly in the 25–44 year age group (Blakely *et al.* 2005).

These changing patterns in specific diseases in part reflect societal changes in particular behaviours such as diet and tobacco use (Blakely *et al.* 2005; Shaw *et al.* 2005b). Taking tobacco as an example, smoking rates have changed over time, with generally increasing rates in the first half of the twentieth century and a decline in smoking in the latter part of the that century. In most developed countries (including Aotearoa) this 'epidemic' of tobacco use has been staggered by sex and socio-economic position, so that some population groups have 'peaked' in their tobacco use earlier than others (Lopez *et al.* 1994; Crampton *et al.* 2000; Hill *et al.* 2003; Barnett *et al.* 2005). This staggering is then reflected in the distribution of tobacco-related diseases such as heart disease and lung cancer (Shaw *et al.* 2005b). Such diseases may be initially more common in higher socio-economic groups, but this gradient soon reverses so that higher disease rates are seen in lower socio-economic groups. Eventually the risk behaviour declines in these groups also, with a resultant flattening of the socio-economic-disease gradient.

*Trends in health services*
There is relatively little data on socio-economic changes in health service usage within Aotearoa. Dharmalingam and colleagues used national data to look at changes in avoidable hospitalisation rates from 1980 to 1997 (a period spanning several health reforms) (Dharmalingam *et al.* 2004). They found an overall increase in avoidable hospitalisations, particularly for the very old and the very young. The authors suggest that this trend reflects a decrease in the accessibility of primary health care during the study period. Unfortunately they did not have good data on socio-economic position; however, they found higher rates of avoidable hospitalisations in areas with a high proportion of Māori residents. This ethnic disparity in avoidable hospitalisations did not change significantly over the time of the study.

New Zealand's primary health sector was reformed in the early 2000s with the stated aim of improving access to primary care for disadvantaged population groups (King 2001). There is some evidence that these changes have improved access to primary care for those groups with fewer socio-economic resources (Hefford *et al.* 2005). However, it remains to be seen whether the socio-economic gradient in access is diminished, or whether higher income groups capture a disproportionate share of the gains.

*Trends in the determinants of health*
Trends in household income show New Zealand has become a less equitable society since the 1980s. Comparing the top and bottom 20 per cent of households (by income), the gap between the richest and poorest has increased (Figure 3.17) ( Ministry of Social Development 2005).

Trends in New Zealand's Gini coefficient show a similar increase in inequalities from the early 1980s to the late 1990s (O'Dea & Howden-Chapman 2000).

Taken together, the above data paint a picture of increasing inequalities from the 1980s to at least the late 1990s. Increasing disparities in income are reflected in greater socio-economic gradients in health, including the burden of disease and risk of premature death.

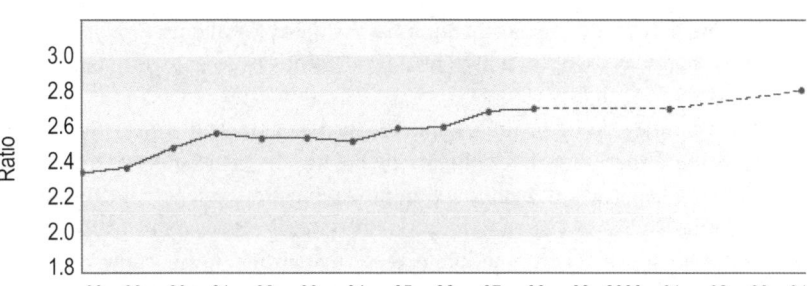

*Figure 3.17: Ratio of disposable household income comparing the 80th to the 20th percentile of households in New Zealand,*[10] *1988–98, 2001 and 2004. Household income is equivalalised for household size and composition. (Data from Ministry of Social Development 2005)*

## What does the future hold for health inequalities in Aotearoa New Zealand?

Inequalities in health are found in every society. However, the degree and nature of health inequality have almost certainly varied with time, and will continue to shift in the future. The patterns of health inequality described here are particular and specific to Aotearoa New Zealand as an economically developed society characterised by capitalism and social democracy. So what is the outlook for socio-economic inequalities in New Zealanders' health? Will health inequalities eventually decline, stay the same or increase? Of course we can't be sure exactly what will happen, but here are a few informed guesses.

First, the distribution of particular diseases in the New Zealand population will continue changing. We have seen that inequalities in some conditions (such as heart disease) are declining, while the gaps in other diseases (such as cancer) continue to increase. This variation is likely to continue as long as lifestyles, behaviours, and values undergo change throughout society. Shifts in the distribution of particular risk factors will be reflected in changing disease profiles and socio-economic gradients. At present, tobacco use is strongly patterned by socio-economic position, but as smoking rates continue to fall over the next 50 years this disparity is likely to diminish. On the other hand, obesity is on the rise and is likely to have a disproportionate impact on those population groups with fewer material resources. These changing risk factor profiles will be expressed in the future distribution of diseases such as diabetes, hypertension, and heart failure.

Second, socio-economic inequalities in health will continue. Regardless of which diseases show a socio-economic gradient – and how steep that gradient is – we will still experience disparities in overall health status, expressed most poignantly in differential mortality risk and life expectancy. The particular diseases that mediate this relationship may change, but the underlying relationship stays the same. To paraphrase Williams (Williams 1997), changes in disease pathways won't change health outcomes as long as the underlying foundations of inequality remain.

Third, the degree of health inequality in Aotearoa will reflect the extent to which the underlying determinants of health are distributed unequally in our society. Disparities in health are an inevitable consequence of differential access to the social and economic goods of society. Provision of timely and accessible health care can ameliorate these disparities, but it cannot remove them altogether: socio-economic gradients exist for non-amenable as well as amenable conditions. We have seen that social and economic policy changes have the potential to widen health inequalities in New Zealand. The challenge for today's decision-makers is whether these disparities can also be reduced.

## Conclusion

As in most developed countries, health in Aotearoa New Zealand is distributed unequally throughout society. This pattern reflects the uneven distribution of the underlying determinants of health – in other words, the tendency for some groups to enjoy greater access to social, economic, and political resources compared with others. These underlying inequalities are played out through intermediary pathways, such as unequal exposure to risk factors for disease and injury, and differential access to adequate health services. The end result of these pathways is a socio-economic gradient in health status, with the most privileged groups in society enjoying the lowest rates of disease and the longest life expectancy, and the least privileged groups having higher rates of disease and disability and shorter life expectancy. Time-trend data suggest these disparities became more pronounced during the 1980s and 1990s, probably as a result of radical changes in New Zealand's social and economic policies. In predicting the future profile of health inequalities in Aotearoa we should consider current social and economic policies, and how these impact on the gap between the most privileged and the most disadvantaged in our society. Socio-economic inequalities and health inequalities are two sides of the same coin.

# 4. Diversity and equity for Māori

## Chris Cunningham

There are more Māori in New Zealand than at any time in our past, and by many measures Māori health and other socio-economic outcomes are more positive than ever before. Yet, as discussed elsewhere in this book, improvements for Māori have not reached those of many non-Māori groups in absolute terms, and many Māori experience persistent disparities in these outcomes.

This chapter describes the increasing diversity of Māori New Zealanders and the inequalities within the Māori population. Reference is made to two research projects being undertaken by Massey University's Research Centre for Māori Health & Development. The first study, *Best Outcomes for Māori: Te Hoe Nuku Roa*, is a longitudinal, random survey of Māori households. The second study, *Oranga Kaumātua: Health & Wellbeing of Older Māori*, is a pair of cross-sectional surveys of older Māori, undertaken at an eight-year interval. In addition the inequalities and equalities in terms of a social, cultural, and economic framework for Māori development will be described.

## Ngā Matatini Māori: The many faces of Māori

Mason Durie first coined the expression 'Ngā Matatini Māori' in 1995 (Durie 1995) in a paper he wrote for the Ministry of Health. In that paper he describes at least three groups of people from Aotearoa New Zealand who all identify as Māori.

> Māori people generally fall into at least three broad groupings. Some Māori are linked with conservative Māori networks. Their children will attend kohanga reo; they will be more or less comfortable on a marae; they will be members of a Māori cultural group or committee; they will speak or understand at least some Māori; they may belong to a predominantly Māori sports team and they will attend tangi.

> Second, there is a group who will have some limited association with Māori society but will be, for the most part, integrated into mainstream New Zealand society. Their lifestyles may not be significantly different from their Pākehā neighbours. But they will strongly resist any insinuation that they are not Māori.

Finally, there is a third group who will not be likely to access Māori institutions nor to take advantage of mainstream services. Their children will have no early childhood education; they may never be part of a marae activity, or visit a library, or belong to a sports club, or attend a Polytechnic ... In effect they will be isolated from both Māori and general society and mainstream services. Yet they will maintain vehemently that they are Māori. And so they are. (Durie 1994a: 10).

While his analysis largely holds true at the time of writing (2006), there is an important and growing fourth group of Māori whom his description does not capture – a group I would characterise as a 'pluralistic elite'. I use 'elite' as a relative rather than absolute term here, because, as other authors have shown, even those Māori who are relatively advantaged are never as well off, particularly in terms of health outcomes, as similarly advantaged Pākehā New Zealanders.

The pluralistic elite group of Māori will be equally comfortable in Māori and mainstream situations. They will have knowledge of their whakapapa, tikanga, and Te Reo Māori. They will visit marae and may enrol their children in bilingual or Māori immersion education. They will be well qualified, well employed, well housed and participate easily in mainstream New Zealand. They will assert their Māori identity on the national and sometimes international stage.

While these four descriptions might capture the experiences of most Māori, what is not so well understood is how Māori move between these 'groupings', or enter and even exit from them. The Māori ethnic group (the combined groupings, or set) is heterogeneous with a number of sub-cultures which seamlessly run into each other. Partly this cultural range is due to the overt influences which result from being a minority culture in a largely western society for more than 160 years. But Māori culture, like other cultures, does not remain static – a memorial to the past; rather it has been developing its own newer course over the past 30 years or so.

## Inequalities and equalities in Māori households

*Best Outcomes for Māori: Te Hoe Nuku Roa*[1] is a stratified, random, longitudinal survey of Māori households which has been quietly developing since 1993 (Te Hoe Nuku Roa Research Team 1999). The survey now covers 650 households with 1600 individuals over six geographically stratified 'cells': Northland, South Auckland, Gisborne–East Coast, Manawatu–Horowhenua, Lower Hutt, and Southland.[2] Since the establishment of this survey in 1993, there have been four waves of data collection at three-yearly intervals. Associated with the study are the development and piloting of a range of whānau-relevant services run by communities.

In broad summary (Te Hoe Nuku Roa Research Team 1999) the study has shown a range of associations with positive outcomes[3] and inequalities in those outcomes. The study has found that access to physical resources, such as land, is low, whereas access to social resources, such as whānau support, is higher and associated with positive outcomes.

Te Reo Māori was found to be in a state of decline, yet a positive attitude towards, and aspirations for, revitalising the language have also been found. Valuing Te Reo Māori *per se* (rather than linguistic ability alone) was associated with positive outcomes.

Most respondents were found to aspire to good health but many are burdened by illness and disability. For many Māori, a choice of a Māori provider is valued, but the study found that this mode of delivery has not yet become universal for Māori and there are wide geographic variations. The study also found that knowledge of, and access to, conventional (mainstream) health services has a key role in supporting health and independence, and is associated with positive outcomes.

In addition the study shows that there is no clear organisational preference for education although opportunities for choice are highly valued. Having the ability to exercise such choices (rather than the actual choice) is associated with more positive outcomes.

Many participants have financial commitments to whānau and Māori organisations. Some manage to make arrangements for their financial futures but many don't, relying heavily on state provision of superannuation. As expected, the study shows that financial independence and literacy is associated with more positive outcomes for individuals and households. Many participants aspire to home ownership, which has increasingly become a priority for Māori. The ability to plan for home ownership is associated with positive outcomes.

A high proportion of, but not all, Māori adults were found to be on an electoral roll (either Māori or general) and most (60 per cent) voted in elections. This finding represents a good measure of social or civic participation, but arguably also of cynicism, with many non-voters declaring the activity a waste of time – for Māori.

According to the study, many adult Māori were involved in leisure activities but few were involved in organised sport. A more sedentary lifestyle, particularly in early to middle-age, is a concern for health outcomes and life expectancy.

A further finding was that children were involved in a range of leisure activities, but few were involved in art or music. The current health status of children was good with conventional (mainstream) health services being the most frequently used. While access was adequate, about a quarter of households reported access problems. Sixty per cent of children had visited a dentist in the previous 12 months. Clearly, accessing services is an area for improvement and one which is equally clearly associated with improved outcomes.

Cultural knowledge is an area of diversity for many Māori. The study shows that knowledge of whakapapa was varied – many knew their waka and iwi (but often not hapu), and most could name at least two generations of their Māori ancestry. Our analysis has found that greater knowledge of whakapapa is significantly associated with better outcomes across a range of indicators.

Adult Māori were reasonably happy with their education although many had had no Māori content in the formal system and would like to have had a Māori component in their education.

## Inequalities and equalities for older Māori

Māori life expectancy is still six-to-eight years shorter than that for Pākehā, and the numerous cultural and whānau roles some older Māori are expected to fulfil causes additional pressure during the last phase of life. This area is an important one for research as many of New Zealand's social policies use age as a criterion for benefits; clearly such an approach disadvantages whole populations with shorter life expectancies. Further, increasing diversity within the Māori population raises the question of how improvements in outcomes are more broadly achieved, and requires a much better understanding of the health and well-being of older Māori.

*Oranga Kaumātua*[4] is a pair of cross-sectional surveys of 400 older Māori, undertaken in 1997 and 2005, which has been designed to assess well-being in the broad sense of the term, including health, material circumstances, cultural well-being, and whānau well-being. The survey uses a network sampling[5] method without trying to achieve a representative sample. A focus is whether older Māori across a range of cultural experience have the same or different outcomes.

The studies give a number of interesting findings. First, older Māori view kaumātuaship as a functioning role, rather than a role which necessarily accompanies older age; some older Māori never expect to achieve kaumātua status. Operating as a kaumātua places a burden on older Māori, and for some it is a considerable burden which can and sometimes does affect their own health and wellness.

Older Māori are very positive about their self-assessed health status, despite the well-known fact that their morbidity and mortality outcomes are poorer than those of their Pākehā peers. This optimism persists in spite of general expectations that ageing necessarily includes increasing frailty. It is only when their physical or mental health affects their ability to operate 'culturally' that older Māori become much less positive.

Contrary to what is perhaps the popular view, fewer than half of older Māori live in a whānau setting; most live alone or as a couple. Few older Māori have made private provision for superannuation or medical insurance, relying heavily on state provision and the contribution of wider whānau.

# Outcomes axes: Towards measurement of intra-ethnic inequalities for Māori

By combining the results from the two studies described above, it is possible to identify four axes of outcome along which inequalities can be measured in a manner sensible to a Māori view: identity, collectivity, human resources, and the Māori estate. Furthermore, these axes of measurement can be applied when interpreting the results of these studies.

A *secure cultural identity* results from individuals being able to access Te Ao Māori[6] and to participate in those institutions, activities, and systems which form the foundations of Māori society. *Collective Māori synergies* represent a community dynamic, where the focus is not only on the position of individuals, but also on community cohesion and the interdependence of individuals, whānau, hapū, and iwi. *Māori cultural and intellectual resources,* especially Te Reo Māori, can be used as a measure of positive outcomes. While the resource itself can be measured, from a community perspective it is *access* to these resources which supports positive Māori development. Differential access to these resources results in inequalities.

The *Māori estate* recognises the Māori worldview, which considers the relationship between people and the wider natural environment (land, forests, waterways, oceans, and air). Reciprocity requires that these physical domains are given due recognition. Again differential access to the Māori estate results in inequalities.

For older Māori, variations in cultural identity, the ability to network with the collective, and access to the broad Māori estate are associated with observed inequalities. That is, there is an implicit requirement to understand the nuances and privileged signals of a Māori worldview. Those who also understand the nuances and privileged signals of a mainstream worldview are potentially doubly advantaged. Those whose cultural access is to the mainstream exclusively tend to have outcomes similar to those of their mainstream peers (of similar deprivation).

# Dimensions of measurement for intra-ethnic inequalities in health

Developed from *Best Outcomes for Māori – Te Hoe Nuku Roa*, Te Ngāhuru (Durie *et al*. 2003a), a Māori outcomes schema, provides a number of indicators relevant to the measurement of inequalities in health. The goals and targets can be expressed in terms of health inequalities as shown in Figure 4.1.

By applying this schema as an analytical lens on the findings of the longitudinal survey, we can see a clear set of processes which support the addressing of inequalities in health outcomes, yet inequalities in 'hauora' require the specific use of a 'hauora lens'. This prospect is elaborated in the following section.

| GOALS | TARGETS |
|---|---|
| Positive participation in society as Māori | Health services are responsive to and actively support the Māori concept of hauora |
| Positive participation in Māori society | Māori are actively involved in the delivery of health and disability support services to Māori |
| Vibrant Māori communities | Māori communities are actively involved in the planning of health services, e.g. through District Health Boards |
| Enhanced whānau capacities | Māori are able to provide adequate care for the population of older Māori; positive assessments of health in Māori terms are measured; multi-generational Māori households exist in greater proportions[7] |
| Māori autonomy | Increasing numbers of Māori-managed and governed health and disability support services |

*Figure 4.1: Goals and targets expressed in terms of health inequalities*

## Understanding health inequalities in Māori terms: Cultural diversity, hauora, and whānau

The relationship between cultural diversity and health outcomes is one that has received little attention for Māori in New Zealand, yet understanding the possible relationship between these two factors is an attractive research question.

While ethnicity and race have been the classical variables for analysis, particularly when comparisons with mainstream New Zealand are sought, there are two major problems that stem from an understanding of the underlying definitions of ethnicity. First, 'ethnicity' as a concept is poorly defined, at least in the minds of those who are most important to any analysis – the respondents. Second, the phenomenon of ethnic mobility across time affects time-series data significantly.

Many of the analyses that have been undertaken in New Zealand rely on a definition of ethnicity principally designed for statistical convenience. These definitions have required mutually exclusive groups, multiple yet prioritised categories, and unqualified self-identity. In many ways some definitions of ethnicity are little more than 'race in disguise'. Some view ethnic identity as an expression of eligibility, others see it as an expression of group membership which is associated with operation within the group. Some see ethnic identity as a political statement that is subject to popularity and the broader political environment. The 2005 general election's emphasis on the 'playing of the race card' no doubt strengthened the identity of some and repressed the ethnic identity of others.

No-one has yet completely accounted for the significant ethnic mobility which is known to occur (Ajwani *et al*. 2003). Such mobility appears to occur for a number of reasons; strictly speaking, the two related phenomena seen are ethnic mobility *and* context effects (Statistics New Zealand 2005). Ethnic mobility is actual respondent desire to change, context effects are more environmental and include the various tools and methods for collection of these data. Mobility can be influenced by the particular questions asked, who is asking the questions, the mode and venue of the interview (responses given face-to-face at a marae may be very different to those in a telephone interview) as well as the broader social environment. It would also appear, from the experience of the Research Centre for Māori Health and Development at Massey University with repeated questionnaires, that many respondents have no precise memory for their previous responses. Further, a small number of respondents 'game' in response to such questions, adapting their particular answer to the situation which faces them. Part of the ethnic mobility phenomenon is the adoption of additional ethnicities rather than the 'loss' of a Māori identity. Thus some respondents who might identify as 'Māori' only, may change their response to 'Māori/Pākehā' on another occasion. Such behaviour, and ethnic identity appears to be a behaviour, makes use of ethnicity as a proxy indicator of culture problematic. Some authors (Pomare *et al*. 1995) have attempted to use 'sole Māori' and 'mixed-Māori' ethnic identities as a possible way of disaggregating the Māori population, but ethnic mobility and context effects make this approach untenable over time.

Both *Te Hoe Nuku Roa* and *Oranga Kaumātua* have attempted to measure cultural diversity as a means of disaggregating or distributing the Māori sample for analysis. A brief schedule of questions, based on extensive qualitative research that has sought to identify a number of cultural indicators for Māori, has been developed. These indicators have not been designed to provide a measure of acculturation in some quantitative manner (differing scores meaning respondents are somehow *more or less* Māori than other respondents); rather they have been designed to illustrate the different expressions of culture among Māori.

In summary, the primary cultural diversity indicators are represented by the seven descriptions which are discussed in the following paragraphs.

### Having 'Māori' as a preferred identity

An interesting result from the *Oranga Kaumātua* study is that not all Māori respondents identify as Māori in every situation. Most respondents will identify as Māori and may sometimes add another ethnic group, depending on the situation. But the high degree of ethnic mobility partly implies that many respondents have no particular memory of the ethnic identity choices they have made previously. In a recent research study undertaken by the Housing and Health Research Programme (He Kainga Hauora), which operates out of the Wellington School of Medicine and Health Sciences (see Chapter 12 by

Philippa Howden-Chapman and Sarah Bierre), the same questionnaire was administered by the same researchers in the same environment but nine months apart, and 18 per cent of Māori respondents made different choices in each interview. As all the respondents were Māori, they tended not to drop Māori as one of their ethnic groups, but tended to add or drop identity with other ethnic groups (Pākehā, European or Pacific).

## Valuing Te Reo Māori

A strong cultural view is represented through valuing Te Reo Māori *per se* (rather than linguistic ability alone). Successful Māori education initiatives such as Te Kohanga Reo and Kura Kaupapa Māori have been supported by parents and grandparents who may have no ability with Māori language but who value its use and knowledge base for their mokopuna. Māori children who are raised in an environment where they are supported to become bilingual often have other positive influences on their broader development and consequently better outcomes.

## Being on the Māori Electoral Roll or an Iwi Register

Being registered on the Māori electoral roll is seen as an expression of political view and possibly social participation. Being registered with an iwi is seen as an expression of affiliation and membership, and some Treaty settlements and Māori networking initiatives such as Tuhono[8] have resulted in an upsurge of registrations. Iwi affiliation is not exclusive; individual Māori and whānau may affiliate to several iwi. Within *Te Hoe Nuku Roa* some 15 per cent of Māori would not identify with an iwi.

## Identifying with a Māori political view

In recent times the emergence of a viable Māori political party has motivated many Māori to express a strong Māori sovereignty view. However, some Māori have always expressed a strong Māori political view, often privately, but increasingly in a public way.

## Having a high level of comfort on marae

Marae have become reasonably ubiquitous in New Zealand with an increase in the number of urban marae, which are often built with the blessing of mana whenua groups. While migration to the major urban centres has meant that home marae are at some distance, the urban marae have filled the void for many. Although relatively few would live on the marae, for major hui, tangi, and other events, marae still play a valuable role. Some, but not all Māori who live away from their own rohe (iwi-specific geographic area) take the opportunity to return 'home' occasionally.

## Contributing to whānau dynamics through knowledge and associations

Many Māori say that they mainly associate with other Māori, usually whānau members and friends. The *Oranga Kaumātua* study, however, shows that fewer than half of older Māori live in a whānau setting, with most living in a single or couple-only situation.

### Understanding Māori concepts

Many concepts such as manaakitanga, whānaungatanga, matauranga, hauora, and others are seen as critical to a Māori identity.

It is at this conceptual level that an analytical challenge in understanding health in Māori terms is encountered. Hauora is a concept which, while related to the western concept of health, is *not* the same as health. Models that describe hauora are well articulated and feature prominently in many of the strategies and health services in New Zealand, both those delivered by Māori providers and those delivered in the mainstream. Te Whare Tapa Whā, Te Wheke, and Ngā Pou Mana are all models which have been adopted as analytical frameworks.[9]

Yet, an even more challenging issue is that not all Māori wholly subscribe to this cultural (hauora) view; therefore any such framework would run the risk of being invalid as it would be based on the false premise that the Māori difference (from Pākehā) is a homogeneous difference. Much of contemporary Māori culture, as expressed by Māori individuals, households, and whānau, is eclectic in nature, borrowing from a range of influences. While most Māori would understand the concept of hauora, they would also understand the concept of health and move between these concepts as situations, and their own volition, dictate.

It is possible to design an analytical framework premised on health (physical and mental well-being and independence) or hauora (physical, mental, spiritual, and whānau well-being). The reality would appear to be that these concepts are best represented as a set of intersecting circles (like a Venn diagram, see Figure 4.2). Māori are much more likely to be distributed within the circles and, importantly, are relatively mobile within the space. Measures of inequalities have to either take one or other perspective, or be flexible enough to adapt to these intersecting concepts and the mobility of Māori within the space.

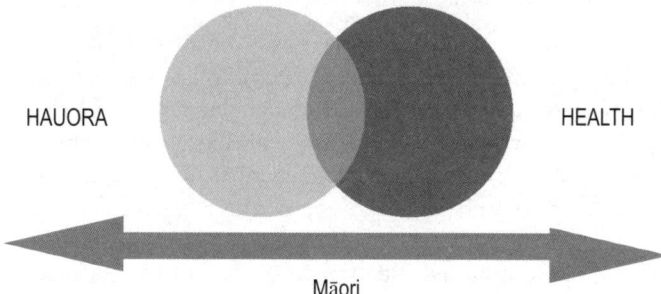

*Figure 4.2: The concepts of health and hauora represented as a set of intersecting circles*

So is there a higher-level framework capable of organising these related, intersecting concepts and mapping the dynamic locations of respondents? And are these relative locations associated with health (hauora) outcomes and inequality? And from whose perspective? These are vital questions for a responsive analysis, and ones which are neither routinely asked nor answered in standard analyses in New Zealand.

### Collectivism and whānau dynamics

Popular wisdom and social research suggest that a distinguishing characteristic of Māori society, when compared with western society, is the focus on the collective rather than the individual. If Māori operate collectively, then what is the most important collective? Three obvious choices exist: iwi, hapū, and whānau, yet it is the whānau structure which seems to have withstood both colonisation and urbanisation (Cunningham 2004).

Contemporary Māori use the term 'whānau' to refer to a range of groups (Durie 1994b; Metge 1995), some rely upon customary whakapapa-based definitions, while others are not based on descent or kinship. Mason Durie (Durie 1994b) defines whānau as:

> more than simply an extended family network, a whānau is a diffuse unit based on a common whakapapa, descent from a shared ancestor, and within which certain responsibilities and obligations are maintained.

However, he acknowledges that the term 'whānau' has been broadened in more recent times to include a number of:

> non-traditional situations where Māori with similar interests, but not direct blood relationships, form a cohesive group (Durie 1994b).

Graham Smith, in 'Whakaoho Whānau Ohanga', defined the whānau as:

> a collective concept which embraces all the descendants of a significant marriage, usually over three or more generations. However, it also refers to the more recent notion derived from its usage in describing a 'group of Māori who may share an association based on some common interests such as locality, an urban marae, a workplace and so on (1995: 23)

Whānau is widely recognised as the basic social structure within Māori society (Ministry of Social Development 2004). It has been used to denote a core group of individuals predominantly comprising three to four generations of family who are intimately intertwined with the wider groupings of iwi, hapū, and waka. Within each whānau, the functions of individuals are defined, with the overall objective being that of reproduction, communal undertakings, and socialisation (Metge 1995; Moeke-Pickering 1996). Whilst the implication of the concept's utilisation and understanding by contemporary Māori is often that of whakapapa linkage (Health Research Council of New Zealand 1998), within the modern milieu of contemporary New Zealand society the term is commonly understood as being synonymous with that of the nuclear family. However, whānau is a concept that extends wider than the traditional nuclear family unit, approximating to what many non-Māori generally understand as the extended family (Ministry of Social Development 2004), and has been expanded still further to refer to any of the following groups: a set of siblings and/or descendants of a relatively recent ancestor, which may or may not include spouses and whāngai; the descendants of a relatively recent ancestor who interact on an ongoing basis; descent groups derived from hapū and/or iwi; a group of unrelated individuals who interact on an ongoing basis; and a group of individuals gathered for the purpose of a specific kaupapa (Metge 1995).

Durie speaks of the distinctions between whakapapa, kaupapa, and statistical whānau (Durie *et al*. 2003b). Whakapapa whānau refers to those individuals with shared ancestry and a common line of descent. Kaupapa whānau is used to describe those individuals 'who may not be descended from the same ancestor but share a common mission and behave towards each other as if they were whānau' (p. 15). Statistical whānau refers to the tendency for many publications to use whānau, household, and family interchangeably. The function of each of these whānau configurations will vary according to the overall purpose of the whānau. Consequently, the exact composition, function and purpose of whānau are largely subjective, making analysis at the level of the small collective – in this case, the whānau – problematic as, to date, little rigorous, quantitative, statistical information has been available on whānau. Another Māori word for family, although little used, is 'whamere' – literally a transliteration of the word 'family'. While promoted as a means of distinguishing a Māori nuclear family from a customary, extended Māori family, this term has failed to gain any significant usage.

Contemporary definitions of whānau extend beyond the descent group. In this context the model of whānau (that is, the values and obligations that underlie whakapapa-based groups) is transported into non-whakapapa-based groups. The term whānau is used to express group members' commitment to one another and perhaps to a shared purpose.

*Te Hoe Nuku Roa* and *Oranga Kaumātua* both provide an interesting insight into the operation of whānau and the relationship with health (and other) outcomes. The following trends are evident. First, whānau based on descent or blood ties are highly valued by most Māori, and most Māori identify as being a member of such a whānau. Kaupapa-based whānau are seen as valid but this is a much less popular form. Second, fewer than half of all older Māori live in a whānau setting, and most live in a couple-only or single situation. For those older Māori in rural and provincial areas, it may be that extended whānau have moved for employment and/or education purposes. Third, young Māori report that when seeking advice on their future careers, they do not talk with whānau, whereas Pākehā young people rate families as significant sources of advice (Cunningham *et al*. 2005). Fourth, while whānau may contribute to the resource base of some individual members, contributing to the broader whānau sometimes places particular pressure on some members – notably on older members who may have their retirement or leisure time eroded by support activities ranging from undertaking cultural roles on marae to childrearing their grandchildren.

## Equity and diversity

Research undertaken with Māori from a Māori philosophical basis in partnership with communities is helping to illuminate the workings within the Māori cultural/ethnic group. Clearly an understanding of the strengths and weaknesses of Māori-specific processes, and the known associations with outcomes, ensures interventions can be designed from a relevant basis. The research shows that economics, cultural diversity, access to networks, intergenerational transmission, and experiences of ethnicity are each major contributors to inequalities within the Māori ethnic group.

Health inequalities between ethnic groups cannot be totally reduced to economic position; variations are due to more than just material disadvantage. However, within a single ethnic group, economic position is one significant determinant of inequality. Further, dimensions of cultural diversity can be seen to be associated with variation in access to networks, services, and information, with a resulting effect on health outcomes.

One critical network for Māori is the whānau, which, while still highly valued as an operating institution within Te Ao Māori, is increasingly losing its importance for some, particularly older Māori. The descent or whakapapa-based whānau is still preferred, although kaupapa-based whānau are effective support structures for some. Another critical network is the mainstream, in particular health and education services. While Māori-provided solutions increase choices and produce relevant outcomes for some, the lack of universal provision coupled with geographic variation means the mainstream will remain an important source of support for most Māori.

Educational and economic inequalities can be passed on from generation to generation. While multi-generational whānau can operate effectively for many Māori, not all Māori can access such whānau. Parents' experience of education, particularly the lack of focus on things Māori, creates the desire for different options for their children and grandchildren. Perceptions and experiences of ethnicity are also important and influence the ways in which Māori may experience health.

Although Maori are numerically stronger than we have been, we are also more diverse in terms of social structure, individual experiences, and expectations than ever before. A clear evidence-informed understanding of the strengths of developments around a range of kaupapa is leading, in turn, to a range of health-related interventions within both the Māori-stream and the mainstream.

# Part Two
## Understanding Inequalities

# 5. A historical perspective on the politics of health care

Michael Belgrave

Social inequality and health outcomes are only partly connected to the effectiveness of the health system or to health policy itself. Good health outcomes, improvements in morbidity and mortality rates, are more likely to be influenced by the availability of nutritious food, by the quality of housing, by levels of household income, and even by the level of inequality within a particular society. This understanding is fundamental to the debate over the social indicators of health outcomes, as is the assumption that broader social and economic forces may be more influential on these outcomes than any actions by government. In any period, health policy is subject to wider policy objectives. Historically these policy objectives have included encouraging self-reliance; strengthening the 'race'; providing security for families; and participation for citizens or rights for consumers. Although realising any of these objectives has been constrained by economic challenges, the objectives themselves reflect the social and economic conditions of the period. Understanding these objectives and the values underpinning them gives us an overview of what is possible and what is more difficult at any particular time. This chapter focuses on the relationship between the development of health and social policy in the past, and the impact of this relationship on the present. It looks at the way that changing technology in health provision has interrelated with the key popular and political objectives which informed policy debate at a particular time. It argues that earlier debates have echoes in the present and as such provide both constraints on and possibilities for dealing with the causes of social inequality today.

Through the twentieth century, the health system achieved a key role in New Zealand politics. Governments were increasingly called to account for their management of the delivery of an ever more expensive and complex system for delivering personal health services and population-based health care to the electorate. While health may have been important, the priorities given to particular health issues in popular political culture, and how politicians responded to them, changed dramatically depending on the current issues facing the health system and the general policy framework prevailing at the time.

We cannot understand the current system for delivering health care without appreciating its history. For over a century in New Zealand, there has been a public health department, local hospital boards which have incrementally taken broader funding and service responsibility, and primary health professionals such as doctors, dentists, and pharmacists. This institutional heritage has a continuing impact on contemporary health policy. The separate provision of mental health services in the past, for instance, has cast a long shadow over the integration and funding of the care of those with mental illnesses (Brunton 2001).

The current administrative framework for providing health care in New Zealand has its origins in the Hospital and Charitable Aid Act 1885, which created local elected hospital boards, and in the Social Security Act 1938, which formed the basis for state funded hospital treatment (Cheyne *et al.* 2004). While public health provisions were adopted in a more piecemeal fashion, the key legislative initiative was possibly the Public Health Act 1920, which followed the devastating 1918 'flu epidemic (Dow 1995; Rice 1988; Rice & Bryder 2005). Despite these aspects of structural continuity, the policy objectives of health spending have changed considerably over time as medical technology has developed, as popular understandings of good health and illness have changed, and as the purpose of the welfare state and the values that underpin it have evolved. In different periods, the emphasis given to the needs of special groups, identified as disadvantaged, compared with the pressures to meet the universal needs of the general population has varied. This would be of historical interest alone, if current values and health policy objectives were creatures only of the present. They are not. This chapter argues that understanding the current policy environment involves an appreciation of the debate between the prevailing values and objectives underpinning contemporary social policy, and the values and objectives of previous policies. Such an appreciation may assist in understanding the potential to narrow inequalities in health outcomes and address the hurdles in the way. Policy development can be seen as a response to two interconnected but distinct discourses: one about the role of the state and social policy, and the other about the risks to the health of society and individuals. How these debates unfold has significant implication for current attempts to improve health outcomes by reducing the level of social inequality in New Zealand society.

## The transformation of health policy from charity to protection from risk

First we turn to debates over the role of the state in social policy. The development of New Zealand's welfare state, and the position of provision for health care within it, can be categorised into a number of periods. In the nineteenth century there was an emphasis on individual and family responsibility and a deliberate lack of state provision except in quite constrained circumstances. The prevailing economic philosophy of *laissez-faire*, although being challenged in the late nineteenth century, sought to contain state support for the disadvantaged. Despite the reforming rhetoric of Seddon's liberals in the 1890s, they were far from generous, and the origins of the welfare state lay not so much in this period but in the era that followed, when concerns about ill health and disability were seen as threatening to the whole viability of European society in New Zealand (Oliver 1977; Oliver 1979; Tennant 1979). Fears of population decline and a weakening of the race contributed to an expansion of services aimed at improving health outcomes for children and for mothers (Mein Smith 1986). This concern was based on biological notions of the detrimental effect of disease on society generally. In this period, the risk was not just to individuals, but to a collectively conceptualised idea of race.

These ideas laid the foundations for more comprehensive provision for need in the late 1930s by establishing a range of largely pro-natal and public health services and by extending popular understandings of the state's social responsibilities. The first Labour government's welfare state had its roots in the social engineering that preceded it, but was less bound by biological notions of society which emphasised heredity, and instead idealised the social environment of a nuclear family as the means of achieving public good. New health services, with a focus on personal health care rather than public health, were heavily subsidised and aimed at producing not an ideal race but a society of ideal families (Belgrave 2004). The next period, beginning in the early 1960s, replaced the ideal family with a participating citizen as the primary objective of social policy. In this phase, rights to health care stood poised between the right to participate in society, which at least suggested that there was an ideal society, and the growing importance of individual choice. With the neo-liberal reforms of the late 1980s and early 1990s, the ideal of social citizenship was replaced by that of the consumer and consumer choice. Finally, the last period that we consider is the third-way approach of the post-1999 Labour-led governments, leaving aside the question of whether that government's health policies marked a substantial break with what had gone before.

Pandemics, epidemics, and the public panics they engendered have also been important drivers of health policy. The bubonic plague scare of 1900 provided the impetus for the establishment of a public health department, although doctors had been calling for such a measure for some time (Dow 1995). In 1920 a new public health act was the direct result of the mortality rate and disruption of the 'flu epidemic, while later in the 1920s a maternal mortality scare had a major influence on the development of maternity services and the medical control of midwifery (Mein Smith 1986; Rice 1988). In the same decade, concerns over the medical fitness of recruits to World War I would find their way into new programmes for dealing with children's health, such as health camps and dental services (Bryder 2003; Tennant 1994). Each of these threats and panics, with its mixture of crisis and opportunity, has played its part in the development of public policy and an increasing sense of state responsibility for both personal and public health issues.

From the beginning of the twentieth century, increasing scientific knowledge and the rising status of the hospital and the medical profession contributed to a popular belief that disease could be conquered, but this also drew increasing attention to medicine's shortcomings (Belgrave 2000; Shorter 1991; Smith 1993). Faith in science made the obvious threat of epidemic diseases more problematic. Knowledge of the origins and transmission of infection, particularly cholera, typhoid, and tuberculosis, gave scientific authority to the suggestion that the medical profession and the state could improve life expectancy and reduce the impact of disease. Poverty, dirt, poor housing, and overcrowding were not simply the responsibility of the poor, as they had been in the political economy of the nineteenth century, but became the sources of plague and pestilence for everyone. Improving the health conditions of the poor could be increasingly seen as a dire necessity for maintaining the well-being of the better off.

These ideas were also significantly influenced by the primacy of biology in nineteenth-century science and popular culture. The debate over evolution and its impact on the developments of eugenics and social Darwinism allowed much of the consideration of public health issues to be focused on society as an organism, which in turn allowed a holistic view of the health needs of individuals and the community. Individuals were understood as organically linked to each other and therefore if one part were affected by illness there would be consequences for all. Ill health amongst the poor, and poverty itself, were thus seen as issues detrimental to the well-being of society as a whole.

For much of the early and mid-twentieth century there was a convergence between concerns about public health and personal health, in that there was a common, even communal, sense of risk. One of the most significant influences underlying the belief that individual ill health could have significant detrimental impacts on society as a whole was the fact that, between the 1860s and the 1940s, increasing knowledge of microbiology produced no effective tools to counter infection once it had taken hold, at least not until sulphonamides became widely available after 1935.

A sense of threat from an unseen and newly discovered world made the prevention of disease more significant than its cure. Ill health as a result of infection had a more direct effect on people of all social classes than it does today. Tuberculosis, for instance, a major killer throughout the nineteenth and early twentieth centuries, appeared to have only partial respect for social status, intellectual ability or even wealth (Smith 1988). Although this lack of discrimination was far from random, tuberculosis still found its way into élite households. Finding the means of preventing ill health and infection, and for treating those who were infected, could be described as having positive advantages not only for the individuals concerned but for the community as a whole, because all could see themselves as potentially in the same situation. This understanding of disease and treatment lent almost complete support – the doctors excepted – to the moves to establish social security in health care with universal, largely free, access. The doctors, led by the dogged president of the British Medical Association (New Zealand Branch), J.P.S. Jamieson, were also committed to a form of social security, but preferred a two-tiered system whereby they could charge the wealthy directly (Hanson 1980; Jamieson 1941). The compromise was a single-tiered and therefore universal system, but one where the private market for primary health care was retained. As a result, plans for a population-based system of primary health care were shelved. Expenditure followed the individual patient choice of practitioner and was not directed to those most in need.

The doctors' success was a testament to the status of scientific medicine and their control over it. In little over a century, doctors had achieved a moral, administrative, and legal authority over health care, at least partly as authorities on the new scientific knowledge of disease and managing the threats to infection. Although sometimes at odds with their colleagues in private practice, heath department doctors dominated health policy. Doctors managed all major health institutions and had greater influence over the elected hospital boards than in the past. Licensing legislation gave them control over almost all other professions and semi-professions in the health sector, and alternative practitioners barely existed (Belgrave 1991). In a more socially conforming age, health professionals were able to ensure substantial compliance from patients, leading to high levels of participation in vaccination programmes and in children's dental services, without the state needing to coerce parents. This reliance on the authority of doctors in a society where health issues were also rising in popular significance also contributed to high levels of institutionalisation for mental disability and illness, and for physical disability. Social security enhanced doctors' authority over health by undermining any alternative, and therefore unsubsidised, practitioners' ability to compete in the medical market place.

## From charity to good health for all

As the twentieth century wore on, the balance between concern about public health and personal health care shifted dramatically in favour of the latter. This was particularly so after 1938 and the establishment of the social security system for delivering primary and secondary health care. The issue of equality of access to health care for families, the key health objective of the Social Security Act 1938 which introduced the welfare state, shifted attention away from collective race protection objectives to those focusing on the well-being of individual families. This shift represented a middle-class opportunity to obtain the benefits of universal access to state-funded services, reflecting a dramatic change in the role of the hospital. The hospital of the mid-nineteenth century, in urban western societies, had been a place for the poor and was avoided by anyone with the means to provide for their own health care in their own homes. While in the New Zealand system, as inherited from the United Kingdom, élite doctors worked in hospitals, they did so to develop their skills and for the status that it brought, but their paying patients remained outside in private practice. The discovery of anaesthetics, and the development after the 1860s of the modern antiseptic and then aseptic theatre, turned hospitals from poor law infirmaries into the universal workshop of doctors. As a result, those who previously would have been treated only in their homes found it increasingly necessary to gain access to the hospital and not simply for surgery, but also for a growing range of services from X-ray to recuperative care.

Few private clinics in New Zealand were able to provide the new technology and the administrative and nursing services at the same level as that available at the growing number of public hospitals. The charitable character of public hospitals, which flowed from their association with the needs of the poor, continued, while the institutions admitted patients from the new middle classes and the élite. This particular development, state provision for the health needs of all, when need was previously associated with poverty, contributed to public acceptance of universal social spending. Hospitals were provided by the state, because the state alone had the resources to do so. Yet people from all social classes needed their services. The state then took on a legitimate role to pay for and provide services for all while maintaining some of the old attitudes to hospitals as institutions of charity and public responsibility.

All of these trends would have an influence on the first Labour government (1935–49), which drew up the model for the first universal public health system in the world. Yet as previously mentioned, in 1938 Labour's intention to introduce a population-based health system that would provide for all was significantly compromised by the resistance of the medical profession. Labour wanted to pay doctors a fixed fee for the number of patients they served. The model was common among Friendly Societies where doctors contracted with the societies to treat their members for a fixed fee per annum and was also applied in the limited scheme for poor patients introduced in Britain from 1911. Doctors generally loathed both forms of medical care and fought to avoid the model being introduced in New Zealand, fearing that they would become mere salaried state servants, losing their entrepreneurial and professional independence. Without the doctors' compliance, however, Labour's health policies could not be implemented. The resulting system, which did not emerge until 1941, had a far greater emphasis on individualised personal health care, and on a micro-economic market for health services, than the Labour government had ever intended. Primary health care was organised and paid for on the basis of individual demand – not overall population objectives. Hospital care was provided without charge, and specialist care was expected to be provided primarily through hospitals. The doctors' ability to use their success in negotiating for patient charges did not lead to a stratified system of health care to any large degree prior to the 1960s. Private hospitals barely survived, public hospitals greatly expanded in size and services, and the state subsidy for primary health care was sufficiently generous to ensure that general practitioners received relatively high incomes from patients in all socio-economic areas.

This emphasis on community health fitted well into the almost universal experience of the baby boom generation. With high levels of fertility and a growing population supplemented by the immigration of young families, particularly from the Pacific, as well as the integration of Māori into the health system after World War II, the health needs of the community appeared to be relatively homogeneous. The heyday of New Zealand's welfare state was based on a particular understanding of health threats prevailing at the time as well as the common needs of a society going through a common demographic transition.

In the welfare state of the 1930s and 1940s, the focus on an idealised family made problematic the health needs of those who did not fit the mould, and these people were less well provided for. Māori and Pacific people were included because their health needs benefited from better housing, higher incomes, and better employment prospects. The welfare state's emphasis on families suited Māori and Pacific needs, if on uncompromisingly western terms. Full employment meant that men and women came in equal numbers from the Pacific and, together with Māori, had high levels of fertility. Both groups' needs for employment, housing, education, and health care were not out of step with those of the majority population, but would become so in the later twentieth century. The needs of single parents and working women were barely acknowledged and those of gays and lesbians not at all. However, perhaps those most disadvantaged were those with physical and mental disabilities. Institutionalisation and social exclusion for these groups possibly peaked in the mid-twentieth century. This trend can be linked to the earlier eugenic objective of isolating 'defectives' from the rest of society and preventing them from passing their defects to later generations, but it was also a means of dealing with a group of people who did not fit into an idealised welfare state. The eugenics aspect of the race protection era would be largely discredited by the use that Nazi Germany made of such ideas, but it should not be assumed that these ideas disappeared completely.

This conservative welfare state, as established in the 1930s, and as it continued almost unchanged through to the 1960s, was based on stereotypical gender roles and saw the basic unit of welfare as the family. Health outcomes were emphasised, not just in provisions for primary, secondary, and tertiary health care, but also in the priority given to public housing and food subsidies (although some of the targets for these subsidies, such as full milk and butter, may seem bizarre today (Steel 2005)). A healthy society was considered the basis of a good society. The biological emphasis of the late nineteenth century had reached its zenith.

## Individualism and health care: A question of rights or consumer choice

In the 1960s the priority of nurturing healthy families was challenged by the increasing importance of the citizenship rights of individuals. In health care, this development also reflected changes in technology. Increases in the use of antibiotics and the growing sophistication of personal health care, driven to some extent by the developing market for drug therapies, further shifted the focus away from public health to personal health provision. Much of this shift was disguised by the egalitarian language of social policy debates during the 1960s and 1970s. Access to good health care became a right of every citizen, but the emphasis on providing an overall healthy society became less important, superseded by issues of personal participation and choice. Community social insurance against risk became subtly less important than, in the language of the Royal Commission on Social Security of 1972, rights to participate in society. From the Hunn report on Māori affairs in 1960 onwards, the special public health measures for Māori, which aimed at raising the health status of Māori families to that of non-Māori, gave way to the objective of ensuring equal treatment of individuals on the basis of civil rights. The urbanisation of Māori left specific health improvement programmes behind in the countryside. In towns and cities, Māori would be left to find their way through the mix of services available to all in the post-1938 welfare state.

Choice played only a small part in the development of health services until the later 1970s, despite becoming increasingly important in the provision of welfare. While in 1941 the doctor's emphasis on personal health care was a triumph for individual choice in the market place, the kind of health care being provided was homogeneous, and choice was limited to the selection of an individual practitioner. Therapies were homogeneous and alternative therapies pushed to the margins if not suppressed. Private hospitals and private medical insurance, all but killed off after 1938, re-emerged slowly following the establishment of the Southern Cross Medical Care Society in 1960 (Fougere *et al.* 1992; Smith 2000). However, the political pressure to improve and extend the range of state subsidised services available to all continued to dominate moves to improve choice in health care. The notion of patient rights was almost non-existent.

By the middle of the 1980s, choice and the belief that need could not be understood on a population basis, but was differentiated by the varied wants of individuals became a leading driver of health policy, as it was in most other areas of social policy. The emphasis on individual citizenship rights, guaranteed by the state, which had underpinned the 1960s and 1970s, readily metamorphosed into faith in individual consumer choice, guaranteed by the market. Health needs shifted from being universally determined by the indiscriminate risk of disease, to being heavily differentiated by ethnicity, gender, and age. The conservative welfare state of 1938 had made clear distinctions on the basis of gender, but in a way that integrated the needs of men, women, and children, under the superior needs of the family. However, by the mid-1980s, attitudes regarding the integrating role of the family gave way to a much more individualistic understanding of need. The cervical cancer scandal at National Women's Hospital in the mid-1980s, the Bill of Rights Act 1990, and the increasing demands that health services be sensitive to the needs of Māori were clear evidence of this new direction. The rights being confirmed were consumer rights rather than social rights. While Māori and women may have been able to assert different needs as a result of these changes, these assertions were on the basis of an individual's rights to choose. The rise of these rights was also paralleled by a declining emphasis on social and universal rights to welfare, housing, and employment. The legitimacy of public health care was further eroded by a breakdown in an earlier unquestioning public confidence in both the state and the medical profession. This alliance had underpinned the welfare state from 1941 by lending scientific respectability to the state and a heavily subsidised monopoly to the profession.

Faith in the market and individualism represented two significant shifts: the first was in the way that community health needs were perceived, and the second was in the changing technology that was available for meeting these needs. The emphasis on patients' rights and consumer choice, coupled with a declining belief that we are all equally subject to the same health risks, undermined political support for state-directed intervention aimed at bridging gaps in health outcomes. A welfare state resting on high degrees of individual freedom and choice made universal participation in public health measures more problematic. New Zealand has rarely legislated to ensure compliance in measures such as vaccination or children's dental care. Such measures have historically proved largely unnecessary, particularly when services were provided through schools. The forces of social conformity generally produced compliance. In recent decades, however, gaining consent from parents for any and every medical intervention has proven a barrier to high levels of participation. In the late 1990s, the National government toyed with making benefit payments dependent on having children immunised, but this was unlikely to have been implemented. Increased levels of poverty since the mid-1980s, the increased transience of those with low incomes, and the increasing costs of services are still more important factors in getting children access to medical services of all kinds.

Once health care became differentiated, involving greater degrees of elective procedures and even allowing for the gradual re-emergence of alternative therapies, along with improvements in medical technology, it was possible to see the needs of individuals as different and linked more to personal choice and lifestyle than to universal threats of infection. The absence of many communicable diseases through immunisation eliminated from popular memory the fear of epidemic diseases. The moral right of society to insist upon universal vaccination was challenged by those more concerned about the risks associated with being vaccinated. The increasing commodification of recreation in the development of a fitness industry made personal trainers an aspect of conspicuous consumption, no less than an expensive car. Many of the new therapies were about easing discomfort rather than providing interventions which had a significant impact on mortality. At this level the question of public support becomes much more problematic.

No longer associated with giving protection from a universal threat, health outcomes now came to be linked with what appeared to be poor lifestyle choices, resulting in ill health due, for example, to obesity, alcohol consumption, lack of exercise, and poor diet. That the illnesses associated with choices were heavily associated with poverty, ethnicity, and even geographic location suggested to many health researchers and social democrats that the underlying cause was social inequality, the reduction of which required substantial state intervention. However, in the 1980s a new breed of individualism with its focus on neo-liberal reform could blame these health characteristics on the failings of individuals making poor choices about their own lives. A re-emergence of neoclassical economics meant that a health system that provided universal support for those who were ill was seen as doing no more than providing perverse incentives for individuals to continue unhealthy behaviour. Their poor lifestyle choices were being rewarded by expensive services provided by the taxpayer. Until the mid-1980s, differentiated needs in social and health outcomes could be categorised as a social problem linked to structural inequality with its source in capitalism or racism. From the mid-1980s, different outcomes were dismissed as evidence of the failure of a state system of health and social service delivery. A reformed health sector would, these reformers hoped, produce the correct financial incentives to encourage healthy behaviour.

The health reforms of the early 1990s reflected many of these assumptions. They were designed to make the whole sector responsive to market forces, by splitting providers from funders and policy-makers, to allow providers to compete with each other. The reforms aimed to provide financial incentives for healthy behaviour, encouraging private insurance, placing user charges on services, and reducing the proportion of funding provided for health care by the state. Creating quasi-markets in health care even became a means of addressing inequalities in health outcomes, since these outcomes were attributed to the performance failures of a state sector that was non-responsive to women, Māori, and Pacific consumers. Turning patients into clients, together with the development of Māori and Pacific health providers, would, it was expected, allow greater participation and greater quality of service.

Despite the neo-liberal underpinnings of these reforms, they were not without supporters from Māori and Pacific groups who saw new opportunities for taking a greater level of control of and participation in health provision (Kiro 2001). The reforms were challenged directly by populist rather than social democratic opinion, crystallising during the 1996 election around the New Zealand First Party campaign of Winston Peters. This populist challenge stressed a return to the universalism of the 1960s and 1970s and was aimed at maintaining the universal principles of middle-class access to the system, particularly for older people. Opponents of the neo-liberal reforms who were more concerned with the impact of the reforms on those finding themselves in increasing levels of poverty, particularly children, were more likely to accept greater targeting of those in need rather than universal provision. This latter approach, advocacy on behalf of the worse off, gained little popular political support. Lower income groups were much easier targets for welfare reform than middle-class and middle-aged users of the health system, and much less able to resist the reforming measures. While issues of cost were important, middle-class consumers benefited much more extensively from services which were free to the consumer than did groups where language, poverty or ethnicity were barriers to access.

Universal services, free to the user, were available in the post-1938 family welfare period, but accompanied by much more limited demands on the health system than is presently the case. There was also a broad consensus about what these services should be. In the decades immediately following the war, popular memories of epidemic diseases and pre-welfare state health standards were still strong. Working class and Māori acceptance of the role of the state in maintaining social and health standards was probably at its peak during the 1940s and 1950s. Even the existence of a working class (in any European understanding of the term) which may have mobilised resistance to the imposition of state-directed welfare policies, welfare officers, and public health nurses has been questioned by some historians (Fairburn & Olssen 2005). Universal services may not have successfully included Māori and Pacific migrants to the same levels as others, but both these groups saw significant improvements in health status over this period. By the end of the century, the free and universal provision of health services was, by itself, unlikely to achieve similar outcomes. In an environment where patient rights are paramount, where social pressure to conform is much weaker, and where all interventions require consent, universal provision cannot be a panacea for social inequality in health outcomes. Poverty, poor understanding of English, limited literacy, and social and cultural isolation all contribute to ensuring unequal participation in universal services, unless groups disadvantaged in these respects are specifically targeted. Aiming to ensure equality of access by eliminating the direct cost of services can accentuate rather than ameliorate differences in health outcomes for different groups.

Yet policy-makers have been clearly caught in a political dilemma in trying to find a balance in health policy between universal and freely available services (for which there has always been strong political support in New Zealand) and those services that are targeted to those with the most need. During the 1950s, the state struck a successful balance between these two objectives, by specific public health policies aimed at improving Māori health alongside 'cradle to the grave' social security measures. Part of the success of these policies lay in the specific health needs of Māori at the time, in the ability to show improvements in health outcomes, and in the lack of attention drawn to the resources going into Māori health. In contrast, where ethnic group outcomes became a priority during the brief flowering of the Clark government's 'Closing the Gaps' policy, the objective of removing barriers between Māori and non-Māori soon became politically untenable. By 2000 the issue of separate funding for Māori had become politically problematic, interwoven with public perceptions of

Māori sovereignty claims and Māori separatism. Even before 2004, when Don Brash's Orewa Rotary speech attacked Treaty of Waitangi-based social policy as 'privileging' Māori, the government had substantially withdrawn from the approach in its public rhetoric, particularly in health. The issue of poor Māori and Pacific health status became subsumed under the more inclusive rubric of population-based health care.

This emphasis on systems of delivery – on health sector reform or on the Treaty of Waitangi and social policy – drew attention away from the more structural problems associated with increasing inequality accruing from the 1980s and at least in part flowing from the socio-economic reforms introduced by the Fourth Labour and Bolger National governments between 1984 and 1993. It is likely that the reforms were directly responsible for greater relative poverty, higher levels of unemployment, and in 1991 dramatic reductions in living standards for beneficiaries (see Susan St John's discussion in Chapter 8; Easton 1997a; Roper 2005). These reforms accompanied an erosion of the foundations of reasonable health standards for those in poverty – in particular, adequate diet and comfortable housing. There were major negative consequences for children, who were in significant numbers within families in poverty. Whether there was any alternative to the reform process is now largely unanswerable, but what is clear is that when this inequality became self-evident in the early 1990s, very little was done to address it directly. Even a decade later, 'Working for Families', the Labour-led government's 2004 budget programme and much delayed commitment to redress the 1991 budget cuts to beneficiaries, has leapt over the needs of those at the bottom to provide relief to the politically more influential middle-income earners.

## 'Third way' health policy: Reconciling past values with present realities?

The current health and welfare system, as it has been re-jigged since 1999, is often referred to as a third-way policy environment. The third way, a term coined to describe 'New Labour's' approach to social and economic policy in the United Kingdom and promoted by Anthony Giddens, describes an attempt to find a balance between two now historical approaches to social policy (Blair 1998; Giddens 2000; Powell 1999). The first, a social democratic tradition, with an emphasis on state management and control and egalitarian outcomes, had roots in the Fabian movement which favoured gradualist and evolutionary socialism (Cheyne et al. 2004). The other way rested in neo-liberal social and economic reform, which emphasised markets and community and individual responsibility and denigrated state planning. The third way was an attempt to find a compromise between these apparently mutually exclusive approaches. The neo-liberal approach was the predominant policy paradigm for the 1980s and much of the 1990s and had its origins in classic nineteenth-century liberalism, while social-democratic ideas marked a compromise between earlier liberal and Marxist approaches.

Third-way governments have not replaced the major structural reforms of their neo-liberal predecessors, but they have softened the emphasis on the market. State planning and coordination of services have re-emerged as priorities and the rhetoric of cooperation and partnership has replaced that of competition and consumer choice. Third way governments are less suspicious of policy advice from health and other professionals. In New Zealand, this has allowed for the recombining of large social policy ministries, such as health and social development, once clinically divided into separate funders, providers, and policy-adviser organisations (Easton 1997). Perhaps the most important aspect of third-way administrations is their belief that the state should direct increasing resources at social problems rather than use tax cuts to allow consumers to make their own choices.

The coming to office of a Labour-led government in 1999 has, with some cause, allowed commentators to draw similar conclusions about a third-way approach for public policy formation in New Zealand. Helen Clark's administrations have reinvigorated the idea of state planning and placed less emphasis on market forces to resolve problems in the delivery of health care, but at the same time have made no attempt to replace the contract-based framework for delivering health care introduced by the Bolger National government. The current government has also fallen short of many aspirations of Labour's supporters for a broader attempt to reduce social inequality. New Zealand Labour's approach to equality has fallen short even of Britain's New Labour, in failing to set clear targets for the reduction of child poverty, for instance (see Susan St John's discussion in Chapter 8). These failings may be seen as particularly severe given that the government has been blessed with high levels of economic growth and substantial surpluses. There have, however, been some achievements, with moves towards population-based health services and considerably increased funding for health care. A renewed focus on prioritising public housing has also responded to two of the key indicators of poor health outcomes, overcrowding and poor quality, in particular damp and cold, housing.

## Conclusion: Can our egalitarian past help deal with inequality today?

In outlining the key characteristics of each of the above periods, care should be taken not to idealise any particular approach to health policy. Even more importantly, it should be evident that even if one period had key characteristics that were valuable, the combination of social policy objectives and values, and the technological and scientific approaches to health risks were unique to that period and therefore cannot be replicated. There were clear benefits in terms of health outcomes in the deliberate attempt by the state to reduce social inequality in the middle decades of the twentieth century, but these decades were also marked by the denial of patient rights, high levels of institutionalisation, and understandings of need that idealised a middle-class Pākehā family over all others. The level of public consensus on these objectives was high, and hardly replicable half a century later in very different social and economic conditions. Egalitarian policies, in themselves, did not ensure lower levels of social inequality. They were accompanied by a widespread trend towards greater social equality among developed countries in the post-war world (Esping-Anderson 1991).

Past policy does not readily sit on the shelf to be picked up at later times. But it does have influences in much more contemporary ways. The values and objectives of these earlier periods still have political influence through debates on social and health policy, at least partly because of intergenerational differences in the perception of need. Those who brought up families in the 1950s and 1960s have retained many of that era's assumptions about health policy, while very different views can be found in their baby-boomer children and grandchildren. Above all, the parents of the baby boomers identify more strongly with state provision of health care and see risk as more universally shared, a view held even more firmly as they become older and need services more regularly. Younger generations have grown up in a period when a century of increasing state social responsibility has been reversed.

None of the periods discussed has been completely silenced in contemporary policy debates, although some have more credence than others, given the different circumstances of different times. In the period of neo-liberal reform during the early 1990s, loud echoes could be heard from the late nineteenth century, as government sought to divide the deserving from the undeserving and to overcome 'dependency' on the state by attempting to reduce government services and benefits and encouraging self-reliance. Debates about eugenics, a key aspect of the race protection period, have re-emerged due to new genetic technology. However, these debates now take place in an environment that privileges individual rights and choice, giving them a new context.

The race protection period introduced many of the services that persisted through the twentieth century, such as dental clinics and health camps, but their purposes changed as the policy objectives for the state changed. Good teeth and healthy boys and girls were linked to concerns about military manpower in recruiting as well as to the belief that Anglo-Saxons in the South Pacific needed to protect themselves against a rising flood from the Asian deluge. But towards the end of the twentieth century, these services were focused on benefiting individual health care and strengthening families.

Vaccination, antibiotics, international regimes to contain pandemics, and improved diet and hygiene have limited the number and virulence of such threats, even encouraging a return of popular suspicion of national immunisation programmes. Smallpox may have been eradicated and polio confined to a handful of cases; however, AIDS, SARS, bird-'flu and resistance to antibiotics are reminders that epidemic and pandemic diseases will re-emerge and could be major threats, even to the developed world. The popular interest surrounding Geoffrey Rice's new edition of his history of the 1918 'flu epidemic in New Zealand was substantial, at least partly due to concerns about bird-'flu in 2005 and the need to draw on historical experience to comprehend the scale of the risk of pandemic today (Rice & Bryder 2005). Such recent concerns bring public health issues to the fore, yet provide narrowly defined debates, with little significant impact on the health system overall.

While populist appeals to maintain and increase the health system's coverage of need continue with some force, they are less based than previously on a consensus on what these needs are and how they should be met. The needs of older people in an ageing society have general appeal – aspiring to live a long and healthy life is a universal objective – but support for such services is tempered by an officially encouraged fear that they will be unavailable to younger generations when they need them.

The diversity in popular understandings of good health continues to increase, with, for example, gay men, Māori women, and those placing their trust in an expanding market for alternative therapy, providing just a few instances of this diversity. Individual need, the consumer's right to choose therapeutic interventions and diagnosis all act as a counterweight to the notion, once more common, that everyone is at the same risk of death, illness, or disability. This sense of risk was once an important feature in giving political legitimacy to attempts to reduce social inequalities of access and health outcomes.

Populist appeal was still able, in the late 1990s, to blunt severely the ability of neo-liberal reformers to use individual choice and diversity to absolve the state from responsibility for health outcomes. Māori have been able to use emphasis on individual consumer sovereignty as a basis for pursuing more collective agendas in the provision of health services. Attempts to privatise and devolve state services in the 1990s led to widespread growth of Māori health providers using contracts with the state to meet what they saw were the collective needs of Māori tribal communities and their members (Kiro 2001). The hoped for flowering of private insurance, to cover all aspects of middle-income health care, never eventuated as increasing premiums, a response to government attempts to contain health budgets, created disincentives for insurance cover. The dependence on expensive, state-funded, hospital services has persisted as the great majority of the New Zealand population remains unable or reluctant to pay directly for these services as they are required, even through private insurance. Universal access to the hospital remains a cornerstone of the welfare state as it has been since 1938, even as the cost has increased, and there is still a high level of public support for such measures. However, the persistence of popular commitment to universalism in health care contrasts with a much smaller commitment to policies to reduce social inequality more generally. Given the influence of poverty on health outcomes, this trend is of more concern. Despite a greater public acceptance of expenditure on the health system, this system, however restructured or reformed, cannot be responsible for reducing social inequality generally. We must look to social policy measures in general with the broader objectives of reducing poverty, particularly among children, of improving housing conditions and improving diet, to see greater declines in disparities between identifiable advantaged and disadvantaged groups in New Zealand society. The historical evidence suggests that however targeted these approaches may be to those most in need, they will succeed best when those better off see that these policies will also have major advantages for themselves or for the society with which they strongly identify and whose overall well-being they value.

# 6. Discourse, media and health in Aotearoa

## Tim McCreanor

Society in Aotearoa is marked by major ethnic and cultural disparities in health and well-being. Inequalities between Māori and non-Māori are deep-seated and well documented in a broad range of domains, including health (Pomare *et al*. 1980, 1995; Ajwani *et al*. 2003); wealth and income (Spoonley *et al*. 1991; Howden-Chapman 2005); and education (Smith & Simon 2001; Hattie 2003). These inequalities are the result, at least in part, of political and bureaucratic practices established in the colonisation of the country by Britain (Sharp 1990; Belich 1996; Durie 2004; Fitzgerald 2004; Cunningham & Durie 2005; Howden-Chapman 2005; Reid & Cram 2005). Popular contemporary explanations of this state of affairs emphasise the responsibility of individuals for their life choices and experiences in ways that match the neo-liberal political climate that has been established over the last 20 years (Kelsey 2002; Witten *et al*. 2003). Such explanations also fit with social Darwinist justifications of the exclusion and marginalisation of indigenous peoples (Goldberg 1993; Smith 1999) that have been central to settler[1] culture here since the early 1800s (Belich 1986; Ballara 1986; McCreanor 1997; Walker 1990a).

This chapter takes the position that such accountings are at best partial and divert attention from the critical role that contexts or environments, particularly social environments, play in the establishment and maintenance of this unjust, exploitative, and unsustainable status quo (Snedden 2005). It is argued that far from being mere words, the ways in which we talk and otherwise communicate about these issues are of central and material importance in creating and maintaining our social orders. The case for this is made by building on research and critical studies that have analysed Pākehā discourse, and particularly mass media discourse, as a key facet of the social environments and representations of Māori and Māori-Pākehā relations. It is also argued that it is insufficient to regard racism as a matter of individual behaviour, and that even in broad definitions which acknowledge institutional and systemic forms of marginalisation based on race, discourse is a key component in the production and reproduction of discriminatory practices.

Despite early observations of health, vigour, and longevity among tangata whenua (Banks 1962; Beaglehole 1968), ideologically, European settlers in Aotearoa arrived wedded to imported racisms (Ballara 1986; McCreanor

1997) such as the 'fatal impact' theory (Adams 1977). This popular notion that indigenous populations would melt away before the superior, civilising mission of the settlers (Moser 1888; Sinclair 1977), was discredited by Māori diplomacy, resistance, and innovation in the nineteenth century (Belich 1986; King 2003), and by major Māori population growth from the beginning of the twentieth century (Sutherland 1940; Pomare 1980; Walker 1990a). Unfortunately, settler acknowledgement that the culture and practices of colonisation are still a key determinant of Māori mortality and morbidity is no longer commonplace. The efforts of academics and commentators such as Moser (1888), Featherston (Foster 2005), and Pember Reeves (1899) to talk Māori out of existence at the turn of the nineteenth century failed, but the diverse practices of representing Māori as inferior and marginal in their own land, remain.

A central tenet of social epidemiology is that the health of populations and population groups are strongly influenced by the environments in which they live (Rose 1992; Marmot & Wilkinson 1999; Wallack 2003). This is a very important stance in a world in which most of the service resources and research effort goes into understandings built around illness and disease in individuals (Antonovsky 1996; Raeburn 2001). Physical features of the world, particularly the quality of the air, water, food, and space that people depend upon are obvious, but often overlooked, factors in determining the health and well-being of people.

Less evident perhaps, and certainly more complex to understand, is the importance of social environments – the interpersonal networks and kin groups that we live within, and the broader social structures (networks of networks) that constitute the communities and cultures that we experience (Bourdieu 1986). These are environments in the sense that they entail the webs of inclusions, opportunities, exclusions, boundaries, resources, accessibilities and so on that influence our experiences, behaviours, interpretations, understandings, and our stories of identity, possibility, and value. They are the contexts in which we experience our lives and, like the physical and atmospheric environments that we occupy, they have strong material and psychological impacts on life chances and outcomes. Billig (1995), utilising Bourdieu's (1986) notion of 'habitus' (the myriad commonplace personal and social practices of communities), refers to the widespread reproduction of and engagement with these social forms as 'enhabitation'. Enhabitation as a broad social process ensures the reproduction of social environments and therefore their role as crucial determinants of personal and collective well-being.

Billig (1995) argues that enhabitation produces cultural forms, such as identity, in at least two distinct ways. 'Hot' practices include processes around issues such as national or regional emergencies, war, and sometimes sporting events, which are actively represented, especially via the mass media, as issues of national pride and importance around which collectivity should cohere. However, Billig is more interested in what he refers to as the 'banal' – the diverse, unobtrusive, everyday expressions of identity and culture that constantly, almost subliminally, remind us of who we are and where our allegiances lie. It is through the combination of these overt, headlining, 'flag-waving' practices, with the mundane, everyday forms, that enhabitation reproduces established social environments.

## Racism and health

Where social environments are positive and supportive of individuals and communities, they are crucially health promoting: the Ottawa Charter (World Health Organization 1986) makes building such environments a central goal of health promotion. However, for many individuals and populations, particularly ethnic and racial minorities, social environments are profoundly health demoting. Causal links between racial and ethnic discrimination (at multiple levels), and the health and well-being of individuals and groups, are increasingly recognised in the international literature (McKendrick & Thorpe 1998; Swan 1998; Williams 1999; Gee 2002; McKenzie 2003; Cain & Kingston 2003; LaVeist 2003; Williams, Neighbors & Jackson 2003). Racism produces direct harm from violence, hazardous low-status work, poor quality housing and physical environments, and reduced opportunities. The resulting societal marginalisation maintains stress at levels which result in multifaceted ethnic disparities in health and well-being over the lifespan of individuals in a wide range of social settings (Marmot & Wilkinson 1999; Karlsen & Nazroo 2003; Krieger 2003).

Biomedical studies have found correlations between blood pressure and racial discrimination in settings such as interpersonal confrontations (Krieger 1990), at work (James et al. 1984; Dressler 1990), and in media representations such as movies (Armstead et al, 1989). In the US CARDIA study, Krieger and Sidney (1996) found elevated blood pressures among American Blacks who respond passively to discrimination compared to those who challenge or resist unfair treatment. Harrell, Hall, and Taliaferro (2003) reviewed the literature on negative physiological impacts created by incidents of racial discrimination and concluded that 'racism increases the volume of stress' experienced, which in turn contributes to stress-related disease.

Experience of racial discrimination has also been shown to be associated with higher rates of mental ill-health (Sanson et al. 1998; Chakraborty & McKenzie 2002; Williams & Williams-Morris 2000) which has major co-morbidity with a range of biomedical conditions (Phelan et al. 2001). A more recent study by Marcovitch (2005) found that fear of racial harassment was negatively associated with self-reported health status.

The US Surgeon General's Office report (US Department of Health and Human Services 2002) reviews a wide evidence base to conclude that racism and discrimination adversely affect physical and mental health, and increase the risk of disorders such as depression and anxiety among minority groups. The report suggests that three general pathways must be considered for improvements in the health of populations that are discriminated against. The first of these is the internalisation of racial stereotypes and negative images, which denigrates individual self-worth and damages social and psychological efficacy. The second is institutional racism, which results in lower socio-economic status and poorer living conditions, in which poverty, crime, and violence are persistent stressors. The third and final pathway is societal racism, which produces stressful events that lead directly to psychological distress and physiological changes affecting mental health.

Karlsen and Nazroo (2003) reviewed multiple studies to conclude that these different forms of racism – personal, institutional, and societal – operate independently and cumulatively to effect negative outcomes on a wide range of health indicators. Nazroo (2003) concluded that racism is an underlying determinant of ethnic health disparities. On the basis of such findings, researchers have advocated for anti-racism programmes as a public health measure (McKenzie 2003) and argued that progress in meeting public health goals requires the elimination of racism (James 2003). Krieger (2003) identified the complex philosophical and political issues involved in treating racism as a threat to public health and concluded that racism is a key field for public good research investment.

## Language as social practice

As suggested in the introduction, it is necessary to contextualise these expanded understandings of racism and engage with the notion of language and discourse as actively producing and reproducing social orders. In drawing upon the notion of discourse, my argument follows that of Potter and Wetherell (1987) and Wetherell and Potter (1992), who maintain that a fundamental feature of language-in-action is that it is profoundly patterned, and that particular interchanges, while unique in themselves, occur within flexible, evolving but nevertheless recognisable, normative boundaries. Discourses are 'relatively coherent ways of talking about objects and events in the world' (Edley 2001: 198) and express a narrow range of expressions of common, socially shared understandings. Discourse operates through the constant reiteration of linguistic resources in everyday social interaction (Billig 1995), in the media and the broad realms of social life. Metaphorically such patterns can be thought of as the building blocks of a conversation as well as the mortar of linkage and conventions of communication, which provide a basis for shared social understanding (Potter & Wetherell 1987; Edley 2001).

Social environments, health promoting or demoting, are inherently discursive and interpretative; in our enhabitation of them we actively create meaning from vast streams of information coming at us in all sensory modalities. We selectively weight and attend to different streams, interpreting inputs according to the established identities and cultures that we are immersed in. The interlocking practices of human communicative and practical activities in social environments produce and are produced by forms of patterning, broadly recognisable as national, community, and personal identity, character, and culture.

Language and text are pre-eminent in the range of ways in which we can communicate and their importance has led critical social scientists (Foucault 1972; Billig *et al*. 1988; Potter & Wetherell 1987; Gergen 1990; Gavey 1989; Fairclough 1995) to advocate the study of such practices, as a topic of major importance in its own right and as a central dimension of any understanding of social orders.

This view is set against common sense and some strands of social scientific theory that argue that language is a neutral medium for the conveyance of information, or in an idiom of anglophones that 'sticks and stones may break your bones but names can never hurt you'; that 'actions speak louder than words'. It is in the interests of established power that discourse, and its active role in the construction of meaning and social reality, is not subject to critical scrutiny because, despite the commonplace and dominant understandings, it is crucial to the ways in which power is manifest through social practices in social orders.

Different language communities with particular conventions and patterns of communication obviously exist between cultures. Within cultural groups, the linguistic patterns also vary over time and between sub-groups (for example with gender, age, and geography), producing tensions and miscommunications. If we deviate too far from the established set of conventions of any particular social or historical location, we risk being misunderstood and/or failing to communicate, which could lead to material consequences.

Similarly, at the level of meaning, there are broad norms that determine the practices of interpretation and comprehension of all facets of lived experience. While some patterns such as traffic rules are explicit and enforced, others (including acceptable sexual conduct) are negotiated and contested. These shared narratives and conventions enormously facilitate social behaviour and the interchanges between individuals because they minimise the need for discussion of social norms. The discourses of everyday talk affect and effect our interpretations of experience, which reinforce the discursive conventions in an ongoing cycle. The normative character of such discourse is recognised in the work of many scholars from Foucault forward, and terms such as 'dominant discourse' (Gergen 1990), 'commonsense' (Billig *et al*. 1988) and 'standard story' (Fish 1980) have been used to describe and analyse it. I have drawn upon the latter in much of my earlier study and re-use it here to capture this sense of these efficient, commonplace ways that we have of addressing, explaining, and rationalising the daily complexities of social life, and rendering the unfamiliar, familiar. A standard story is a loosely bounded multifaceted pattern of talk that is widely recognisable within a culture. It is imbued with a flexibility that renders it capable of being evoked by a few words as well as a more elaborate, extended description.

> While the world given by the standard story is no less a constructed one than the world of a novel or play, for those who speak from within it ... the facts of that world will be as obvious and inescapable as one could wish. (Fish 1980)

Such discursive structures are strongly evident in the ways in which Pākehā talk about Māori and Māori/Pākehā relations.

## Patterns in Pākehā talk

Earlier studies of Pākehā discourses in this field have provided descriptions of a number of identifiable and recurring themes in Pākehā talk about Māori and Māori/Pākehā relations (Abel 1997; Bell 1996; Bell 2004a; Potter & Wetherell 1987; Wetherell & Potter 1992). My own contributions are drawn particularly from the discourse analytic work of the Human Rights Commission database of written public submissions that were gathered following what is known as the Haka Party Incident (Walker 1990b) at the University of Auckland in 1979. This confrontation between engineering students practising an obscene rendition of a haka in preparation for a capping parade and a group of Māori and Pasifika activists who objected to the engineers' behaviour led to arrests and a trial of the activists. The affair was much publicised under newspaper headings such as 'Gang Rampage on Campus: Students bashed at haka practice' and became a watershed of public feeling about Māori/Pākehā relations. The Human Rights Commission advertised for and gathered some 600 public submissions, which became the database for my PhD study, and my analyses of these materials is published in a number of sources (McCreanor 1989, 1993a, 1993b, 1993c, 1996; Nairn & McCreanor 1990, 1991). Here themes from the data are presented in summary form; although rarely used in this form, the themes are nevertheless easily discernible in everyday talk. The first seven of the themes relate specifically to Māori. The remaining themes relate to relations between Pākehā and tangata whenua or to the ideal state of the social order.

### Good Māori/Bad Māori

Māori fall into the two groups, those who fit without difficulty into society and those who can't or won't. Bad Māori are those who reject, resist or fail to meet Pākehā norms or standards. They are mainly young, urban, aggressive, lazy, unemployed, and shiftless. Good Māori are dignified, polite, and mostly passive, rural folk. They are older, humble labourers or modest business or professional people.

### Māori stirrers

A tiny minority of Bad Māori are troublemakers, agitators, radicals or stirrers who are committed to making trouble where none need exist. They are unreasonably demanding and their claims for redress of grievances are unrealistic, selfish, and racist. Stirrers are bent on rousing the quiescent sectors of the Māori population by raising their expectations as to what they should aspire to and receive from the government.

### Māori inheritance

Many people unjustifiably claim Māori identity since they have more 'blood' from other lines of descent and should see themselves as Pākehā. Some individuals do this simply to be able to access various state resources that they would not otherwise be entitled to. Stirrers encourage these identity practices and then use the inflated figures that result to claim a larger share of the common wealth.

### Māori morality

Māori are dishonest and enviously disrespectful of the property of others. They will steal from anyone and cheat on public funding schemes. They have weak moral standards, particularly around sexuality, and poor child-rearing practices. Violence is part of the savage character and Māori men in particular enjoy fighting and actively seek it out. As a result they make tough soldiers and sportspeople but bad citizens and neighbours.

### Māori privilege

Māori have unfair and privileged access to rights and resources unavailable to the rest of society. The Māori Affairs Department, the Waitangi Tribunal, the seats in Parliament, cheap housing loans, their own rugby team, educational supports and quotas, and fishing rights all add up to special treatment which is racist and akin to apartheid.

### Māori sensitivity

Māori are hypersensitive about their culture and its relationship to the mainstream. As a result they are easily offended and seem to have lost their sense of humour when it comes to matters of protocol and preservation of their practices.

### Māori inferiority

The inferiority of Māori culture to that of the Pākehā is obvious and justified by simple comparisons often with the entire composite cultural history of Europe. Māori history consists of myth, art of a few carvings, music of just three or four notes, and the language is dying. The culture cannot compete in the modern world and is dependent upon Pākehā culture for its protection and survival, and ill-fits its citizens to foot it in the modern world. Māori who champion their culture are challenged to forswear cars and television and other commodities to 'go back to their grass skirts'.

### One people

Unless Māori drop their sectarian interests in favour of national unity as New Zealanders or Kiwis, racial tension will continue to grow. Multiculturalism in which minority and immigrant groups add spice and colour to the mainstream society is the preferred model. Biculturalism as a power-sharing model is divisive and dangerous, unreasonably raising Māori aspirations to self-determination.

*Ignorance*

When Pākehā do offend Māori it is usually out of ignorance rather than malice. This often arises because Māori are secretive about their culture or are themselves confused as to what the appropriate behaviour is in particular circumstances.

*Rights*

Equal rights for all citizens is a cornerstone of our democratic society. One person's rights, particularly to the common resources of the nation (and especially the tax dollar), cannot prevail over those of others. Privilege is wrong and anti-democratic.

Study of other data such as media coverage signals the operation of other themes in addition to those arising from the original database. Examples would include the two following themes.

*Treaty*

The Treaty of Waitangi is a flawed historical document of no relevance to the present day. Contemporary New Zealanders cannot be bound by it and it should have no place in our political scene.

*Moriori*

Māori displaced the original inhabitants of this country because they were stronger and more sophisticated. Now the same thing is happening to them but it is just an evolutionary process so they can hardly complain.

This thematic summary, which I am not claiming is exhaustive, serves to orient this discussion of the discursive features of the Pākehā standard story of Māori–Pākehā relations and representations of Māori. As described elsewhere (McCreanor 1997, 2005) there is a strong continuity between the historical and more contemporary usages that supports the claim that these are durable phenomena that are widely understood and used by people wishing to criticise Māori. There is obviously great diversity in the positions adopted by Pākehā citizens on any of these themes and the topic as a whole. Equally, there is considerable contextual flexibility with which arguments are articulated to meet the needs of different situations. Given its obvious resilience and durability, it is argued here that this research-based collage of the discursive resources that can be used to construct the standard story can be a useful tool for understanding the meaning-making at work in particular everyday circumstances. The remainder of the chapter makes the case that this standard story is a key feature of our social environments, and media outputs in particular, and that as such it is an important, modifiable determinant of well-being in Aotearoa.

# Media discourse and race

In Aotearoa as elsewhere, the mass media, both public and private, is an extremely well-resourced and powerful cornerstone institution that wields massive influence on all areas of social life (Rosenberg 2002; Hodgetts & Chamberlain 2003). As the role of media in society has grown, the proportion of what we know from direct (as distinct from mediated) experience has shifted to the point where mass media strongly shape our personal and collective social realities. Analyses of media in contemporary societies have concluded that media are the storytellers, repeatedly confirming and modifying the society's image of itself (Anderson 1991; Hall 2001; Fairclough 1995). In and through these narratives, whether in the factual or fictional genres, we get to 'know' fellow citizens as individuals and groups without ever meeting them directly.

All media storytelling occurs within dominant discursive practices (Fairclough 1993, 1995), the standard stories that include criteria or values that identify events or people as newsworthy. The mainstream media constantly exposes us to depictions that reinforce the established power relations of our society (van Dijk 1993; Nairn 1999). In an earlier publication on this topic, I wrote about the links between media and discourse:

> Media stories both construct and are constructed by those commonsense ideological patterns and associations shared by their audience. The patterns act as boundaries or fields within which the commonsense of a social group can flow with ease and beyond which a speaker's discourse can be expected to meet with hostility or incomprehension. (McCreanor 1993a: 82)

# Mass media in Aotearoa

As with power relations the world over, the media in Aotearoa have played a major role in entrenching and maintaining particular interests at the expense of others (Herman & Chomsky 1988). From the 1840s forward, settler journalists, operating from a worldview that is strongly congruent with the contemporary standard story, constructed the colonial wars as conflicts in which a savage rabble was inevitably overcome by the might and valour of British fighting men (Belich 1986). Such views, along with a general denigration of tangata whenua, were reproduced in the popular press, official accounts, the education system, and other institutions to become an established truth that critical historians such as Belich (1986), Orange (1987), Walker (1990b) and Ballara (1986) have struggled to displace.

Examining the media specifically, Wilson (1990: 49) drew attention to more recent patterns:

> There's nothing [the media] handle quite so badly [as Māori news]. They bungle it in all sorts of ways – playing down big issues (Māori language teaching), missing Māori implications in other issues (immigration), ignoring stories completely (major hui and festivals), quoting people who aren't Māori authorities (Winston Peters or Bob Jones) and neglecting those who are, blowing up negative stories, getting them wrong and denying they did.

These criticisms, which refer to key themes of the standard story (ignorance, Māori inferiority, stirrers, good Māori/bad Māori), fit within the broad framing that the story supports, constructing Māori as problematic in almost every realm. Like the standard story, Wilson's critique emphasises the interlinked negativity and absence of positivity – the powerful, constructive contributions that Māori have always made to our social order are ignored or minimised (Ramsden & Spoonley 1993; Walker 1990b). Pākehā concepts and discourses of race relations pervade media constructions of issues involving Māori. Selective reporting of negative issues, reliance on non-Māori sources, and preferential use of race labels creates and sustains a distorted view of Māori (Corner 1995).

In a comprehensive study that highlights ways in which the media determine what and who is news, McGregor and Comrie (1995) found that stories about Māori issues made up only 5.5 per cent of their total television and radio sample and that journalists relied overwhelmingly on Pākehā news sources for 61.7 per cent of stories. Māori sources were used in only 12.8 per cent of the items. Television coverage about Māori was dominated by bad news, often expressed as conflict between Māori and Pākehā.

Abel's detailed analysis of television coverage of Waitangi Day in 1990 identified several themes of the standard story at work, especially the 'one people' and 'stirrers' patterns.

> The 'unity' discourse which referred to the Treaty (if at all) as a symbol of unity … saw the celebrations as moving people closer together and spoke of 'one people', 'our nation'. It described moves for Māori control over Māori resources and development as 'separatist' (1997: 39)

Abel found that the coverage positioned Māori as either 'wild' or 'tame' (good Māori/bad Māori pattern), masking the breadth of Māori support for protests about Treaty grievances. Further, the media focused on the tactics of protest rather than the injustices that stimulated the protest.

Discursive and content analyses of media coverage of a successful genetics research project that had been initiated by Māori demonstrated that the media attributed the achievement only to the Pākehā partner, a genetics research team at University of Otago (Rankine & McCreanor 2004). The stories failed to acknowledge that the Māori researchers had initiated the project, were responsible for the genealogical component of the work that created computational shortcuts that delivered results of analyses long ahead of projections, and were managing life-saving genetic screening projects arising from the research. The major framing of the story combined the 'good Māori/ bad Māori' and 'Māori inferiority' patterns to cast Māori as helpless victims crying out for help from the Pākehā world of science and technology.

Hodgetts *et al.* (2004) studied media coverage of the report *Decades of Disparity* (Ajwani *et al.* 2003), which detailed the range and extent of health disparities between Māori and Pākehā. They found that the coverage encouraged explanations based on individual lifestyle choices, implied that recently created Māori health services were ineffective and sabotaged the report's strong evidence that health inequalities were structurally determined. No journalists questioned the role of societal structures or mainstream health services in the disparities, and media coverage of the debate ignored sophisticated Māori models of health (Durie 2000) in favour of biomedical conceptualisations. Again the framing depicts Māori as victims of their own health practices and cultural inferiority.

Moewaka Barnes et al. (2005) analysed a randomly selected two-week media sample and found widespread media reproduction of the key standard-story themes of 'Māori privilege', 'one people' and 'Treaty', and also found an emerging focus on inter-iwi conflict and depictions of problems with Māori financial probity and disproportionate reporting of 'bad news' about Māori.

On the basis of these and other studies, it is argued here that the media in Aotearoa are inexorably contributing to the marginalisation of Māori as a group. In Billig's (1995) terms they are a crucial component of the broad culture of discrimination that amounts to the habitus of our society. As such, media outputs are an omnipresent noxious agent to which Māori are constantly and serially exposed. As I have written elsewhere (Nairn et al. 2006: 191):

> We have sketched the media contribution to promoting and maintaining Pākehā domination. Critical analyses of media representations of Māori and relations between Māori and settlers have been shown to favour the latter and, in a variety of ways, damage the former.

## Conclusion

The research record demonstrates a deep-seated and ongoing failure of media accountability on representations of Māori. In other settings, similar critique and dissatisfactions have led to movements and calls for participatory or civic journalism (Scammell & Semetko 2000; Wallack 2003), through which media professionals and institutions can be realigned with the needs of broad populations and communities rather than narrow or sectional interests. The Pew Foundation (2005) defines civic journalism and emphasises its potential:

> At its heart is a belief that journalism has an obligation to public life – an obligation that goes beyond just telling the news or unloading lots of facts. The way we do our journalism affects the way public life goes. Journalism can help empower a community or it can help disable it.

Key developments in the media in this country, particularly the rise of iwi radio stations, the emergence of Māori television, the re-emergence of Māori print media (particularly in magazine format), and a growing cadre of Māori journalists, illustrate what can be achieved. However, the established media are lagging far behind in this work and actively undermining the gains.

Following Krieger (2003) and Nazroo (2003), it is argued here that it is necessary to conceptualise racism in all its forms as a crucial public health issue. Among all the banal practices that contribute to the exclusion of Māori, we need to focus on media performance as a key vector in the transmission of these damaging social practices. In this country, the relative decline in the health status of Māori (Ajwani et al. 2003) is a major priority. Public health approaches that seek changes that can lead to social and physical environments that are health promoting rather than demoting are therefore a crucial tool in rebuilding Māori health.

In conclusion, while there is a large body of evidence already to hand about the negative role of the media in health disparities, combined research-monitoring and social transformation projects that aim for empowerment and inclusion of Māori in national and community life are crucial. A research-based platform to guide media reform toward realising its potential through positive and holistic representations of Māori and Māori-settler relations is needed. The development of more Māori-controlled media to contribute toward the improvement of Māori health and well-being is also needed. In turn, these reforms and projects are vital components of the Māori development and participation which will constitute a socially just, productive, and vibrant nation.

# 7. Does poverty affect health?

### Brian Easton

**M**uch of the international research on the social determinants of poor health in rich countries focuses on the effect of socio-economic status (SES) – a composite of such things as occupation, education, and housing conditions. However, there is not a lot of SES data readily available in New Zealand, so household disposable income, adjusted for household composition ('equivalised'), is sometimes used as a proxy because it can be directly influenced by policy instruments. The two variables need not correlate well, for household income varies both in the short term and over the life cycle, while SES is largely for an adult's life. Lifetime income would be a better indicator of SES than current annual income, but again there is not much data available.

What the international research shows is that there is an 'SES gradient', in which those with low SES experience higher morbidity from respiratory and cardiovascular diseases, ulcers, rheumatoid disorders, psychiatric diseases, dementia, a number of cancers, and so on. Often those at the bottom of the SES scale have life expectancies five to ten years shorter than those at the top of the scale (Wilkinson 2005). Part, but not all, of the differences can be explained by differences in access to health care and by 'unhealthy life styles' such as the consumption of tobacco and excess alcohol, lack of exercise, and obesity (all of which might be addressed by conventional health care and health promotion policies). Even so, there remains a significant residual which cannot be so readily explained.

The search for alternative explanations has paid much attention to the social environment, perhaps intermediated through economic and psychological channels. However, in rich countries there is not a lot of evidence that income has a direct effect on health, even though – as we shall see – the poor tend to be sicker. Unlike those in much poorer countries, the affluent nation's poor would appear to have sufficient to purchase healthy food, adequate clothing, reasonable housing, and so on (Sapolsky 2004, 2005).

For instance, today's sickness benefit for a married couple in New Zealand is about 5 per cent more in value, after adjusting for consumer price rises, than it was 50 years ago (and the beneficiary is likely to be entitled to more supplements). Yet there are foodbanks today, while there were none in

1956. The simplest explanation is that real wages (wages adjusted for price changes) have risen about 55 per cent more in the period. In principle, a host of other adjustments should be made, such as for households now earning two wages but paying higher rates of taxation, but the basic conclusion is that the beneficiaries are relatively poorer and find it more difficult to cope.

This is not to argue that had they more income, they could not improve their consumption for a healthy life style, or that they spend their income wisely. (The same is largely true for those with greater affluence.) At issue is that by itself it would appear that income is not a determinant of health, although it is a correlate. Once the minimal resources are available to sustain a basic level of health, absolute levels of income seem unimportant in determining health.

In recent years it has been proposed that the intermediating channel is stress. There is a substantial biomedical literature which has established that individuals are more at risk from stress-sensitive diseases – which include many of those listed above as being associated with the SES gradient – if they fall into one or more of five groups. In the first are those who feel they have minimal control over stressors, and in the second are those who feel they have no predictive information about the intensity of the stress. The third group are those who have fewer outlets for the frustration caused by the stressor; the fourth interpret the stressor as evidence of circumstances worsening; and those in the fifth group lack social support for the duress caused by the stressors (Sapolsky 2004, 2005).

While there has been less research to test the hypothesis, it is plausible that the poor are subject to greater disease-inducing stress than those further up the income scale. This is not to argue that others do not suffer stress, but that they have better opportunities to cope with it (in terms of the points made in the previous paragraph) than the poor. An intriguing insight is that while the objective state of being poor appears to adversely affect health, the subjective state of feeling poor seems even more important (Adler 2003), in which case the notion of relative poverty levels becomes very relevant. Many of the stresses – such as those of inferiority feelings because of low spending power – do not go away just because of a general rise in income. Thus the downside of having a low income in a rich country involves different mechanisms to that in a poor country. The notion of an absolute poverty line is no longer relevant, while relative poverty is. It is possible that the observed connection between income inequality and poor health is an effect caused by stress (Kawachi & Kennedy 2002). The most probable channel is that the lower a household is in the social pecking order, the more likely that it is to experience stress.

Low household disposable income is not the only route to sickness that the stress hypothesis identifies. Other economic phenomena cause health-damaging stress. The best studied is unemployment where it is clear that psychological and financial stress puts the unemployed person and her or his partner at risk. More generally, early life experiences, social exclusion, work, and lack of social support as well as unemployment have all been identified as sources of health-damaging stress (Wilkinson & Marmot 1998).

# Changes in the New Zealand income distribution: 1980s to mid-1990s

New Zealand household income inequality increased sharply in the late 1980s and early 1990s. Figure 7.1 shows that the shares of the bottom four quintiles of (equivalised) household disposable income fell between 1987 and 1997, with the top quintile gaining the 3.3 percentage points the remaining 80 per cent lost.

On some comparisons the increase in inequality was the greatest in the western world over the period (Easton 1996).

Unfortunately in 1997, in a cost-saving measure, the New Zealand government replaced the annual household survey, from which the income shares were derived, by a triennial one, so it is more difficult to discern trends afterwards. However, Figure 7.1 indicates the likelihood that the bottom two deciles continued to lose disposable income share, the middle one made some gains but did not recover back to its 1987 level, while the upper two deciles seem to have had a share increase. If so, inequality continued to increase after the mid-1990s, although the following section argues that it may be due to different causes.

Why did the changes in the late 1980s and early 1990s occur? Aside from the complication of the business cycle, three groups of reasons have been considered. In the first group are the economic reforms involving sweeping liberalisation of the economy (increased use of the market mechanism) from 1984 to 1993. Changes in tax and benefit (and other welfare) policies make up

| YEAR | QUINTILE | | | | | INCOME |
|------|--------|------|--------|------|------|--------|
| (Sep or Dec) | Bottom | 4th | Middle | 2nd | Top | ($2004) |
| 1987 | 10.3 | 13.7 | 18.3 | 24.3 | 33.3 | 23 500 |
| 1988 | 10.2 | 13.5 | 17.7 | 24.0 | 34.7 | 23 300 |
| 1989 | 10.0 | 13.2 | 17.6 | 23.6 | 35.6 | 23 300 |
| 1990 | 9.9 | 12.6 | 17.7 | 24.1 | 35.7 | 22 700 |
| 1991 | 9.7 | 12.3 | 17.3 | 24.2 | 36.5 | 21 500 |
| 1992 | 9.5 | 12.2 | 16.0 | 24.2 | 37.3 | 21 600 |
| 1993 | 9.5 | 12.4 | 17.1 | 24.3 | 36.7 | 21 000 |
| 1994 | 9.8 | 12.3 | 16.7 | 24.0 | 37.1 | 22 000 |
| 1995 | 9.9 | 12.6 | 17.3 | 23.9 | 36.3 | 22 400 |
| 1996 | 9.3 | 12.1 | 16.9 | 24.4 | 37.3 | 22 600 |
| 1997 | 9.6 | 12.1 | 17.3 | 23.9 | 36.6 | 24 300 |
| 2000 | 9.4 | 12.0 | 17.2 | 24.3 | 37.2 | 24 600 |
| 2003 | 9.1 | 11.9 | 17.5 | 24.7 | 36.8 | 25 800 |

*Figure 7.1: Shares of household equivalised disposable income by household quintile. (Source: Perry 2005)*

the second group, and in the third group are the fundamental changes in the structure of the economy arising from technical change and globalisation (the external impact of those forces which are integrating the world economy).

Obviously all the explanations had some effect, but a careful analysis concluded the dominant impact came from policies that cut income taxes of the rich – tax cuts that were paid for by higher income taxes on the poor, cuts in social security benefits, and cuts in other government services (Easton 1996, 1999).

This is not to say that the other effects were unimportant. Unemployment peaked at 11.1 per cent in March 1992, although the percentage at a point in time can be misleading. In the 57 months between October 1988 and June 1993, 754,312 sought work by enrolling on the New Zealand Employment Register (Department of Labour 1994). To give some idea of this magnitude, those who registered as unemployed in the period represent about 47 per cent of the average size of the labour force over the period, or around 10 per cent of the labour force each year when the average rate of unemployment at any point in time was 8.7 per cent. This overestimates the likelihood of being unemployed because of inflows (from school leaving, returning to work, and immigration), and underestimates it insofar as not all unemployed registered.

Whatever is the true figure, it would appear that a high proportion of the labour force experienced unemployment in the period. Those who enrolled more than once are counted but once in the above total. In fact over 45 per cent were enrolled at least twice, and 2.1 per cent more than five times. This suggests that at least 21 per cent of the labour force experienced repeated unemployment in the four-year period, and 1 per cent experienced it on five or more occasions. The average number of enrolments was 1.8 times for non-Māori, and 2.2 times for Māori. The average cumulative duration on the register was 59 weeks – those who identified as Māori averaged 69 weeks. The register does not pick up all the labour market churning, but suggests it was substantial in the period.

However, because the stress was substantial, it was more evenly spread than at first one might have expected. Similarly, while the liberalisation resulted in people both suffering and benefiting, there is a tendency to focus on the big losses. For instance, substantial reductions in levels of protection of the clothing industry resulted in job losses, but the price of the now-imported clothing fell for the population as a whole. Did those individually small but widespread gains offset the large losses to a small set of workers? Or – and perhaps this is more relevant – for each individual, did the myriads of small benefits from the ending of protection in many industries offset the one (or more) big employment losses?

If they did not, was there a particular social group of New Zealanders who were privileged because they received the benefits and were not affected by the downside? When we look at the available data – inadequate though it may be – we can conclude that those on high incomes benefited not from the change in their market incomes but from the marked reductions in income tax they paid. It turns out that many of the rich also suffered – from a loss of wealth, perhaps following the sharemarket crash, perhaps because they too lost benefits from the protection their investments had enjoyed. Equally, there were those on modest and low incomes who would have been better off from the changes, once the terrible transition of high unemployment had worked its way through, except they found themselves paying higher income taxes, or receiving fewer benefits from the state.

This account keeps to the conventional distributional approach, which largely ignores any economic growth and looks only at distributional shares. But in the six years from 1987 to 1993 average income per head fell. (See the final column of Figure 7.1.) The distributional impact was such that real income fell for the bottom four household income quintiles, but remained (roughly) constant for the top quintile, because the tax cuts offset the fall in their market income. Falling incomes are a further source of stress (although again there is considerable churning).

## Changes in income distribution after the mid-1990s

There is no need to report the details of the distributional policy changes which occurred after 1996, except to note that there were both progressive and regressive changes, but none were of the redistributive magnitude of the earlier period. Because of the data gaps, it is also harder to assess whether there have been major redistributional changes since 1996. However, there seems to have been a tendency for increasing inequality, but this time the bottom two quintiles lose more and the top two (or three) quintiles gain more. This suggests a different redistributive mechanism from that of the previous decade (see also Dixon (1998) for more clues).

There is a vigorous debate about the extent to which the forces of globalisation and technological change are modifying the income distribution of rich countries. It can be only sketched here, beginning with a simplified account of how globalisation may impact unfavourably on the rich country's income distribution. Figure 7.2 characterises the economy by quadrants, dividing it into a tradeable and non-tradeable sector (the tradeable sector is exposed to overseas competition, and the non-tradeable is not) and a skilled and unskilled labour force.

|  |  | ECONOMY | |
|---|---|---|---|
|  |  | Tradeable sector | Non-tradeable sector |
| **Labour force** | Skilled |  |  |
|  | Unskilled | *Hollowed out?* |  |

*Figure 7.2 The structure of a modern economy*

It is the tradeable sector/unskilled labour force quadrant (in the bottom left-hand quadrant) which appears to be 'hollowed out' as simple manufacturing was relocated offshore (particularly to East Asia). The most evident example is demise of the textile, clothing, and footwear industry. There will still be unskilled jobs in the tradeable sector and also in the non-tradeable sector (janitors, for example, will be needed in high-tech food-processing works as well as in rest-homes). However, one would expect that major job losses in the hollowed-out quadrant would reduce unskilled wage rates elsewhere. Unskilled wage rates are low, and wages are an important component of low-income households (see below). Such changes may have contributed to the increased inequality that appears to have been occurring in the late 1990s. The effect of the hollowing out from globalisation is, therefore, increased income inequality, unless there is an upgrading of skills in the labour force.

Broadly the same story applies for technological change except that the (relative) reduction in unskilled jobs is the result of technical change favouring skilled jobs (and it is unnecessary to make the tradeable versus non-tradeable sector distinction, since the technological change can occur in either sector or both). Again, unless there is sufficient upskilling of the labour force, there will be downward pressures on unskilled wage rates and increased household inequality.

## Who are the poor households in New Zealand?

I now report some research Suzie Ballantyne and I did using the Household Economic Survey (HES) for the three-year period covering financial years 1994/5–1996/7 when the HES included questions on the respondents' recent utilisation of health services together with a subjective assessment of their health status, as well as socio-economic variables such as income and expenditure and personal characteristics (Easton 2002; Easton & Ballantyne 2002).

Our work involved detailed econometric analysis, with considerably more care taken in the application of the household equivalence scale, which adjusts for household composition, for housing (since outlays are different for those who own their houses and those who rent), and for the choice of poverty line. The following tables are based upon the Michelini equivalence scale, income econometrically adjusted for housing circumstances, and a poverty line based on the benefit datum line of the Royal Commission on Social Security (1972), although using other assumptions will not markedly change the broad conclusions.

Figure 7.3 shows the proportion in poverty and the proportion of the poor by household type. While the highest incidence of poverty is among households consisting of a single adult with children – as is frequently commented upon – they make up only a sixth of the poor. In contrast, households with two adults and children have less than half of the poverty incidence of the single-parent households, but make up more than twice those numbers. This illustrates the danger of focusing on solo parents and ignoring the vast majority of the poor,

| | Proportion in Poverty | Proportion of the Poor |
|---|---|---|
| Adult not in labour force | 4.6 | 1.6 |
| Adult in labour force | 2.6 | 0.4 |
| 2 Adults, neither in labour force | 6.0 | 3.5 |
| 2 Adults, 1+ in labour force | 4.0 | 4.4 |
| 1 Adult with 1+ children | 38.7 | 16.3 |
| 2 Adults with 1 child | 13.9 | 7.6 |
| 2 Adults with 2 children | 18.2 | 16.7 |
| 2 Adults with 3+ children | 21.5 | 18.0 |
| All 2 Adult-with-children households | 18.4 | 42.3 |
| 3 Adults without children | 7.2 | 8.0 |
| 3 Adults with children | 22.8 | 23.5 |
| In households with children | 21.9 | 82.1 |
| In households without children | 5.5 | 17.9 |
| ALL | 14.2 | 100.0 |

*Figure 7.3: Poverty by household type. (Source: Easton & Ballantyne 2002)*

| | Proportion in Poverty | Proportion of the Poor |
|---|---|---|
| Pākehā | 10.7 | 58.5 |
| Māori | 23.7 | 19.9 |
| Pacific Island | 33.4 | 11.8 |
| Asian | 26.3 | 9.8 |
| **ALL** | **14.2** | **100.0** |

*Figure 7.4: Poverty by ethnicity. (Source: Easton & Ballantyne 2002)*

who are children and their parents, most of whom live in two-adult homes. Households with children contain over four-fifths of the poor.

Figure 7.4 looks at the poor by ethnicity and shows the same pattern of differences between proportion in poverty and proportion of the poor. Non-Pākehā poverty is higher than Pākehā poverty. Yet almost three-fifths of the poor are Pākehā (because there are a lot more of them).

Similarly, Figure 7.5, which cuts the data by housing tenure, shows that renters have the highest incidence of poverty, but that over half of the poor live in their own homes.

|  | Proportion in Poverty | Proportion of the Poor |
|---|---|---|
| Rent | 27.3 | 47.4 |
| Own with mortgage | 13.5 | 37.5 |
| Own without mortgage | 6.0 | 15.0 |
| Rent free | 1.2 | 0.1 |
| **ALL** | **14.2** | **100.0** |

*Figure 7.5: Poverty by housing tenure. (Source: Easton & Ballantyne 2002)*

It is messier, but it can also be shown that the poor households are more likely to receive market income (wages) than to depend on benefits. (Nevertheless beneficiaries with children are more likely to be in poverty.)

In summary, the most common poor New Zealand household is a couple with children who are of Pākehā ethnicity, who own their home with a mortgage, and depend upon wage income. There are other groups who have higher incidence of poverty, but because they are smaller they do not involve as many people.

There is a tendency for poverty rhetoric to emphasise single-parent households, ethnic minorities, renters, and beneficiaries. The reality is that while a household with any of these features is more likely to be poor, the poor are more likely to be mirror images of the characteristics. The policy implication is that poverty eradication involves working on a broad front rather than targeting minority groups. If there is a typical poor household, it is one which contains children.

## The location of the sick in the income distribution

The particular advantage of the years the study used was that respondents were asked to rate their health status on a scale of 'excellent ', 'good', 'fair' or 'poor' health. Very few categorised themselves at the bottom, so we combined 'fair' and 'poor' into a single category. Some 8.6 per cent of the population were in this lowest category. Note the health rating is self-reported and subjective, although self-reported health ratings are regarded as a useful prospective measure of population health status (Idler, Leventhal, McLaughlin *et al.* 2004).

Again there is an apparent paradox in the results, for the sickest are more likely to be in the middle quintile than the bottom quintile of the overall household distribution (Figure 7.6). However, an examination of the characteristics by age and gender shows that the poorest in each category have the highest incidence of poverty (Figure 7.7). The old are the sickest – over half of those in the 'fair' or 'poor' categories are aged over 65 – but they are not as poor as the young. As far as poor health is concerned, age is a more important determinant than income. Even so, within age groups, those in the lowest income quintiles tend to be the sickest. The gradients vary (and are erratic, presumably because of the low numbers involved) and they seem to be

|  | HOUSEHOLD INCOME QUINTILES | | | | | ALL |
|---|---|---|---|---|---|---|
|  | Bottom | 2 | Middle | 4 | Top |  |
| ALL | 21.7 | 25.3 | 25.5 | 16.3 | 11.2 | 100 |

*Figure 7.6: Percentages of total who rate themselves as having 'fair' or 'poor' health. (Source: Easton & Ballantyne 2002)*

|  | HOUSEHOLD INCOME QUINTILES | | | | | ALL |
|---|---|---|---|---|---|---|
|  | Bottom | 2 | Middle | 4 | Top |  |
| Under 15 Female | 7.4 | 3.6 | 2.9 | 3.1 | 1.2 | 4.5 |
| Under 15 Male | 5.8 | 5.8 | 3.4 | 3.0 | 3.1 | 4.7 |
| 15–64 Female | 19.7 | 11.0 | 8.7 | 7.2 | 3.9 | 7.9 |
| 15–64 Male | 10.2 | 8.3 | 7.4 | 4.2 | 3.8 | 6.2 |
| Over 65 Female | 42.5 | 29.4 | 27.5 | 22.3 | 21.2 | 26.5 |
| Over 65 Male | 40.2 | 29.8 | 25.2 | 21.3 | 19.4 | 25.5 |
| ALL | 9.3 | 11.0 | 11.0 | 7.0 | 4.8 | 8.6 |

*Figure 7.7: Incidence (%) who rate themselves as having 'fair' or 'poor' health. (Source: Easton & Ballantyne 2002)*

stronger for females than males. This in itself constitutes a puzzle – perhaps the females are under more stress.

What the gradients suggest for those under 65, is that health levels in those in the middle three household quintiles are much the same. But poor health is markedly more common – typically about double – for those in bottom quintile households. The top income households tend to have fewer members who are in inferior health. Does their income enable them to purchase better health care? Do they have less illness-inducing stress? It cannot simply be that those adults with poor health tend to sink into lower income groups because their earning power suffers, since children who are sick also tend to be in lower income households, even though their sickness is less likely to reduce family incomes.

## Conclusion

This chapter has focused upon a set of propositions, which may be summarised in five main points.

The first is that in a rich country poverty (i.e. a low material standard of living) probably does not directly impact on health, but does so indirectly through stress which income differences generate.

Second, the increase in household inequality in the period of the late 1980s and early 1990s was more due to changes in tax, benefit, and government spending policies than it was to market liberalisation. However, market liberalisation increased stress on New Zealanders.

Third, there is some evidence that income inequality may be increasing, due to factors such as globalisation and technological change.

Fourth, the most common poor New Zealand household is a couple with children who are of Pākehā ethnicity, who own their home (usually with a mortgage), and who depend upon wages for their main income. There are other groups who have higher incidence of poverty, but because they are smaller they do not involve as many people. This means that effective poverty eradication involves working on a broad front rather than targeting minority groups.

Fifth and finally, illness does not correlate well with income, unless age is controlled for. The sick in New Zealand are the elderly, although it has been argued that policies aiming to reduce poor health in the long term need to target those with low incomes and low in the socio-economic status hierarchy.

The policy conclusions might be that while there is a socio-economic (SES) gradient on health status, services whose purpose is to provide health care to individuals need to give more consideration to the age of the local population. However, the international research evidence suggests that where services are aimed at raising the health status of the entire population over the long term, SES effects appear to be important.

How to target by SES effectively is another matter, especially as it is not the same as income (or even lifetime income, although that would give a better correlation). It seems likely that reducing income inequality may help – especially perceptions of income inequality and/or its importance. But it may also be possible to address some of the stress channels directly. Certainly it makes sense that any policy change needs to be accompanied by an audit of what stress the policy will generate and to what extent people who are already stressed will be able to deal with any further stress burden.

# 8. Child poverty and family incomes policy in New Zealand

Susan St John

The rise of the children's movement in New Zealand and internationally reflects not only the increased awareness that children have unalienable rights as citizens but also a growing appreciation that a failure to invest adequately in children carries high long-term social and economic costs. Child poverty is a complex problem defying simple measurement. Its symptoms are manifested in New Zealand in many ways such as in a high incidence of third world diseases such as meningococcal disease, whooping cough, rheumatic fever, bronchiolitis and pneumonia, high school transience, failure to learn, hungry children, foodbanks, and child abuse (Child Poverty Action Group 2003; St John *et al*. 2001).

There are no easy or quick fixes to child poverty, and improving income alone is not an adequate measure of the success of poverty reduction policies. Nevertheless income is widely implicated in well-being outcomes for children (Duncan 2006). An obvious contributing factor to the growth and severity of child poverty in New Zealand has been the neglect of preventative measures aimed at supporting family incomes (St John 2004). The New Zealand government is now seeking to remedy that by improving the disposable income of families with children through its Working for Families policies and it will monitor such policies with income measures:

> There is a strong rationale for using an income approach, at least as a key component in a measurement regime: current income is a reasonable indicator of the consumption opportunities available to a citizen; and income support is one of the most powerful instruments that a government has at its disposal for its poverty alleviation and resource redistribution goals (Perry 2004: 23).

The crude poverty figures based on disposable income alone clearly show that the economic position of New Zealand children sharply deteriorated in the early 1990s and Figure 8.1 confirms that despite the strong economic growth of the early 2000s, a large number of children, at least one out of every five, were still existing at the margins of society in 2004.

For the past 10 years Child Poverty Action Group (CPAG), have focused attention on the impact of the neglect of the family income assistance system. During the 1990s New Zealand fell far behind countries like the UK and

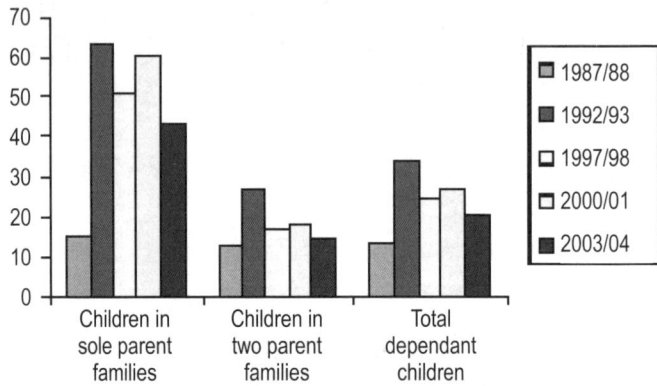

*Figure 8.1 Proportion of children below the poverty line\* 1988 to 2004.*
*\*This is not an official poverty line, but one of those used by the Ministry of Social Development. It is 60 per cent net-of-housing median equivalised family disposable incomes (benchmarked to 1998 median) (Derived from Perry 2005)*

Australia, let alone the Scandinavian countries, in supporting families with children (Stephens *et al*. 1996). It should have been easy to make the case for substantially increasing child benefit-type payments yet it proved surprisingly difficult to get any action on this, or even attract political attention to the issue (St John 2004). It was not until the 2004 budget's Working for Families package that there was any substantial attempt to boost family incomes. This package offered no immediate relief, however, with assistance being phased in over three years from 1 April 2005 to 1 April 2007. Another boost for working families was promised by Labour in the run-up to the election in September 2005, but unfortunately the needs of the poorest children who were not in 'working' families were ignored (St John & Craig 2004).

While the significant real redistribution to low income working families is welcome, the poorest children's needs have been subordinated to the prevailing wisdom that work is the only way out of poverty. There is no doubt that secure, full-time, adequately paid work is fundamental to the security and well-being of most families and is the ideal to be strived for, but 250,000 children currently live in families dependent on a welfare benefit. For most of these families, full-time work is not possible, regardless of the size of work incentives. This chapter turns the spotlight on the poorest in this group, whose relative economic position has continued to deteriorate, with worrying implications for child health outcomes.

## The emergence of child poverty in New Zealand
Many factors have driven the alarming increase in child poverty as shown in Figure 8.1. Notable are the benefits cuts of 1991, the tax cuts of 1996 and the introduction of the Child Tax Credit, the lack of price indexation

of Family Support, the explosion in housing costs, the casualisation of low wage employment, the greater exposure of families to social hazards such as drugs and gambling, and the generally more time-fractured nature of family living. Poor children in New Zealand have largely been politically invisible and it has been very easy for policy-makers to ignore them. The University of Auckland's 2004 winter lecture series 'Trading in our Children's Future' focused on concerns about child health in New Zealand. It was, unfortunately, reminiscent of a similar winter lecture series, 'Status of Children', which was held in 1991. The author's contribution to the 2004 series was a disconcerting echo of a lecture she delivered 13 years ago. One of the illustrations put up in 1991, was a cartoon in which the politician is saying to Ruth Richardson, the then Minister of Finance, 'This budget is going to hit everyone except little children, Ruth.' She replies 'By Jove you're right. I forgot all about them' (see below).[1] Perhaps the cartoonist intended the deep irony?[2] Of course, the 'mother of all budgets', as the 1991 budget was dubbed, in fact entailed a serious but overt attack on the living standards of little children. If children's well-being had been the focus in 1991, and policy had been audited from a child's point of view, the mother of all budgets would never have seen the light of day. If Working for Families had taken a child-focused approach, it might have been differently named and would have placed far less emphasis on work as the solution to child poverty. The income distribution (after allowing for taxes and benefits) has widened since the early 1980s as shown in Figure 8.2, which charts the changes in real disposable income for households, arranged in tenths of the distribution (adjusted for household size). The top tenth of the distribution has dramatically improved its position, with significant overall real gains to the top half of the distribution. The lowest four deciles, where young children are disproportionately located, have all lost ground.[3] This data tells only a partial story as it takes no account of the soaring cost of housing for poorer households nor of the large capital gains reaped in the housing market by those in the top decile.

The economy was particularly buoyant in the first five years of the new century, and families should have been getting their heads above water. Indeed, the data used in Figure 8.2 show that between 1982 and 2004 middle and high income groups gained significantly, but the bottom fifth's incomes

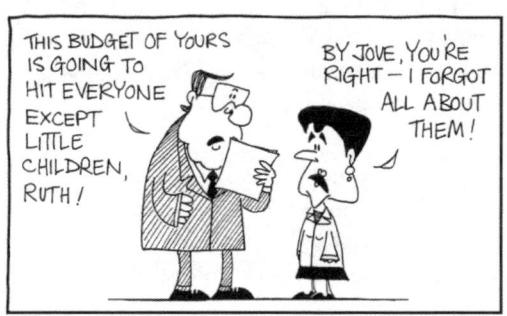

% change

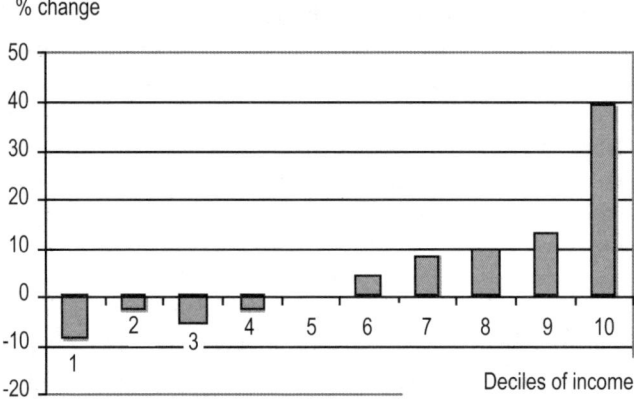

*Figure 8.2: Percentage change in average household equivalent disposable income by household decile, 1982–2004. (Source: Mowbray 2001; updated Statistics New Zealand 2006)*

hardly moved in real terms. It can be surmised that low wages have managed to negate the employment gains for this group. As well, Family Support remained virtually unadjusted for nine years until 2004, with low but steady inflation seriously eroding its purchasing power. In addition, debt repayments, rising interest rates, higher energy costs, and higher rents impact more severely on the lowest income groups, reducing the actual money families have left to feed their families. Thus, despite the so-called good times, it is understandable that the demand for food parcels by families at many of the major foodbanks in New Zealand continued to rise (Wynd 2005). At the Auckland City Mission, record demand continued into 2005, as shown in Figure 8.3. These food parcels are not just the stop-gap tin of baked beans. They are serious attempts to provide sufficient food for an entire family for three to four days. The increased demand is not because of poor budgeting or life skills; rather, it directly reflects a lack of income and an accumulated debt. The neglect of the needs of those in the lowest income deciles over a long period means that an increase in income alone cannot immediately repair the accumulated damage. Families with inadequate incomes run down their assets and often must resort to high interest loans to cover normal expenses. They frequently owe money to Work and Income New Zealand (WINZ) that must be repaid. There is thus a danger in thinking that a mere inflation catch-up in child payments is all that is required to reduce the demand for foodbank services.

## Measuring child poverty

The definitions and measurement of poverty have spawned vast academic efforts and can be highly controversial. Poverty lines pose conceptual and practical measurement problems, but are nevertheless a necessary part of the

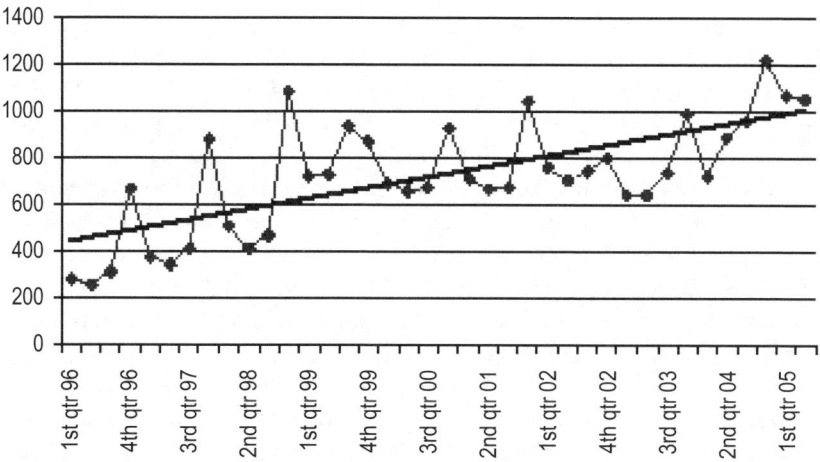

*Figure 8.3: Quarterly Auckland City Mission figures showing number of food parcels given out, 1996 to 2005. (Source: Wynd 2005)*

measurement of the impact of policy changes (Perry 2004).[4] It is important that relative poverty lines are used, because children experience poverty in relation to the standards of living of everyone else. However, using relative poverty lines does pose some perceptual problems: rising median incomes may increase relative poverty numbers while the absolute living standards of the poorest may not be getting worse. Nevertheless lack of material things enjoyed by peer groups can result in social exclusion, alienation, and ultimately poor health. Merely providing the poor with sustenance sufficient only to meet immediate needs is not appropriate in a developed country that seeks to maximise the productive potential of all its citizens. Thus, as advocacy groups have argued in the United Kingdom, a mix of absolute and relative measures is probably the best approach. Preferably these measures would be implemented after housing costs had been met, and would be supplemented by surveys of perceived hardship. Poverty may be judged to be unambiguously falling only when it is falling on all measures of poverty (Dornan 2004). In 1999 in the UK, Prime Minister Tony Blair made a promise: 'Our historic aim, that ours is the first generation to end child poverty forever … it's a 20-year mission but I believe it can be done' (Blair 1999). Since then, much attention has been paid to family incomes and poverty lines. Billions of pounds have been spent on improving weekly supplements, based on the level of parental income and numbers of children, and paid as tax credits through the tax system. The aim has been to reduce child poverty by a quarter by 2005, a half by 2010, and eliminate it by 2020. This policy is beginning to bear fruit, but it is clear that it is a tough road and much more has to be done if child poverty is to be eliminated by 2020 (Dornan 2004).

In New Zealand, specific targets for child poverty reduction have not been formulated. Official recognition of the existence of child poverty first came in 2002, with a promise that it would be 'eradicated' (Ministry of Social Development 2002), but to date no timelines for its eradication have been produced. It was not until the 2004 budget that specific policies to improve low family income emerged, with Prime Minister Helen Clark proclaiming in the budget 2004 speech from the throne that the Working for Families package 'is the biggest offensive in the war against child poverty in decades'. The 2004 budget projected a decline in child poverty by 2007, making it clear that attention would at last be given to monitoring poverty levels. The 2007 target was based on assumptions such as a 100 per cent up-take of the Working for Families package, and an economy that neither slips into recession nor experiences higher inflation. Accordingly projections show that by the 2007/8 financial year child poverty will be significantly reduced. Indeed the 2004 budget projected a 30 per cent reduction. This was based on a poverty-line measure of 60 per cent of the before-housing-costs median disposable family income benchmarked to 1998. This leaves one in five New Zealand children in poverty on this measure (Perry 2004).[5] While this represents progress, there is a lot of catching up to do. Moreover, a relative measure based on the current median is likely to show little change as median incomes rose significantly in this period in a growing economy.

Further progress may require the government to follow the United Kingdom's example by committing itself to poverty reduction goals with the ultimate aim of eliminating child poverty altogether. The lesson we can learn from the UK experience is that both political and public support for change is vital, and that full political commitment and a sustained and generous programme of real redistribution to families is essential in order to make substantial progress towards eliminating child poverty. The encouraging evidence from the UK is that more money does make a difference and that child poverty is not inevitable.

## The neglect of family assistance

The history of family assistance in New Zealand has been one of neglect. From the post-war period, when there was a meaningful and universal family benefit, low-cost medical care and affordable housing, New Zealand has increasingly adopted measures designed for the poorest families only. More recently it has introduced an unfortunate degree of discrimination against the non-working poor (Child Poverty Action Group 2002), as discussed below. In 1986 Family Support was introduced as a per-week per-child tax credit based on family income. Also paid was the universal $6 per child per week Child Tax Credit. A one-child family receiving the maximum assistance was entitled to $42 a week. In 1991 the Child Tax Credit was absorbed into Family Support and reduced against joint parental income. Over time, the effect of inflation in reducing the spending power of Family Support was considerable. In a much needed inflation adjustment, Family Support was increased by $20 per child per week in 1996, but $15 of this increase was carved off and renamed the Child Tax Credit (CTC). Children whose parental income was from a benefit of any kind – such as a student allowance, accident compensation, superannuation, unemployment, sickness, and the Domestic Purposes Benefit – were ineligible to receive it.

The prime focus when thinking about the effects of these changes and the implications for health inequalities has to be the poorest children. The severe neglect of family assistance can be demonstrated by analysing the maximum value of family assistance. Only the poorest children get the maximum, so looking at the real value of the maximum assistance over time is a good indicator of how disadvantaged they have become. To illustrate, let us take the example of a one-child, two-parent family on a benefit. In 1986 their combined Family Support and Child Tax Credit was $42 a week. In 2004 their maximum Family Support was just $47.[6] The loss of purchasing power over the years meant that instead of $47, this one-child, very low income family should have been getting $75. Their loss is illustrated in Figure 8.4.

Also shown in Figure 8.4 is the effect of the introduction of the Child Tax Credit in 1996. Around 300,000 poor children were denied $15 of their rightful compensation for past inflation. They got only a $5 increase in their Family Support instead of the $20 given to the 'deserving' children with parents in paid employment. While $15 may not sound much, it is a highly significant amount for families on tight budgets as it can provide the basics like bread and milk. One way to think about it is that families denied the Child Tax Credit have saved the government over $2 billion since 1996. In turn, this implies that

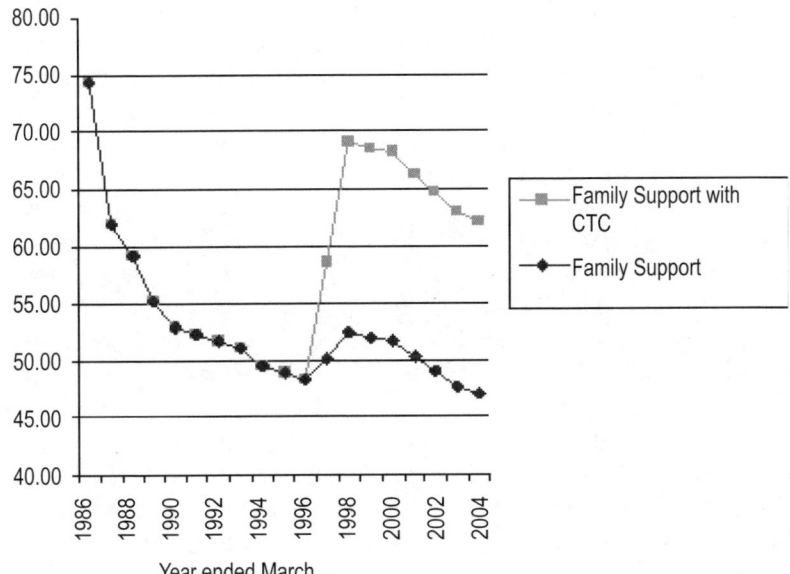

*Figure 8.4 One-child maximum real family assistance 1986–2004 ($2004). (Source: St John & Craig 2004)*

denial of the Child Tax Credit has contributed to high debt levels found among poor families (Wynd 2005).

## The purpose of the Child Tax Credit

The 'work not welfare' mantra, common among politicians on both the right and left, has spawned welfare-to-work programmes in the US and in New Zealand. Indeed it provided the ideological justification for the introduction of the Child Tax Credit in 1996 (O'Brien 2005). The Child Tax Credit, superseded in 2006 by the In work Payment, was a labour market tool, based on the idea that it is important for people in work to be better off than those on benefits. It applied selectively, however, as only those with children were entitled to it, even though it might be expected that childless young people have more need of an incentive to work.

It is possible to show that some parents working for minimum wages are worse off than if they were receiving a benefit, unless there is something like the Child Tax Credit in place.[7] But numerous criticisms of its usefulness as a labour market incentive were mounted (Child Poverty Action Group 2000, 2002; St John & Craig 2004). To begin, the Child Tax Credit rewarded independence from the state, not extra hours worked. It was complex for parents to understand and difficult to administer. The criteria were crude and discriminatory: for example, a child could have been denied $15 per week because one parent is old or disabled, or unfortunate enough to need Accident Compensation for more than three months, or is a student on a student allowance. Rather than a carrot to encourage full-time work, the Child Tax Credit could be seen as a punishment for those who relied on the state for any form of assistance.

Thus the Child Tax Credit must be judged harshly in terms of being a very poor work incentive and because it intensified poverty and contributed to the debt problems among poor families. Compared to the UK and Australia, Aotearoa New Zealand was well out of step.[8] In both those countries per child weekly payments are the same for all children of low-income parents, regardless of the source of their parents' income, just as it used to be in New Zealand before 1996.[9] Both the UK and Australia have a more generous and less targeted approach and both regularly adjust these payments for inflation. In addition both countries have a significant universal component to their family assistance. In Australia, for example, the quasi-universal $21 a week per child is reduced, but only for those on very high incomes.[10]

## The 2004 budget and child poverty

It was disappointing that the 2004 budget promised poor children nothing until April 2005. It was hard to understand a budget that identified a serious problem and then denied any need to deal with it in the current budget year. Figure 8.5 sets out the main changes to family assistance announced in the 2004 budget, and the additional improvements for 2006 announced in August 2005 in a pre-election statement.

| Maximum family assistance | Pre April 2005 | 1 April 2005 | 1 April 2006 | 1 April 2007 |
|---|---|---|---|---|
| **Family Support** | | | | |
| Ist child | 47 | 72 | 72 | 82 |
| Subsequent children | 32 | 47 | 47 | 57 |
| **Child Tax Credit (CTC)** | | | | |
| Each child | 15 | 15 | 0 | 0 |
| **'In-Work Payment' (IWP)** | 0 | 0 | 60 | 60 |
| Per family $ per week | | | + $15 each child for 4 or more | + $15 each child for 4 or more |
| **Thresholds for abatement** | | | | |
| 18% | $20,356 | $20,356 | | |
| 30% | $27,481 | $27,481 | | |
| 20% | | | $35,000 | $35,000 |

*Figure 8.5: Working for Families: Maximum family assistance 2005–2007. (Source: derived from Ministry of Social Development (MSD), Working for Families website http://www.msd.govt.nz/media-information/working-for-families/index.html)*

In April 2005 Family Support was increased by $25 a week for the first child, and $15 for subsequent children with another $10 promised in 2007. On the surface these changes restore the purchasing power of maximum Family Support, but the cumulative damage done by 18 years of diminished purchasing power remains.

Figure 8.6 will be explained more fully below, but the top line shows that by 2007/8 the picture is much improved for those who get the 'In-Work Payment' (IWP). The In-Work Payment is $60 a week, increased by $15 per child for families with more than three children. It certainly boosts the incomes of 'in-work'families, and will have a significant impact on child poverty in low income working families who take up the tax credits, but drives a large wedge between those who qualify and the poorest benefit-dependent families.

## Children in families on benefits

Families who miss out on the work-related payments because of their relationship with the benefit system may appear to have had their Family Support restored in real terms by 2007, as illustrated by the middle line in Figure 8.6, but their actual gain is usually far less. In 2005 the child-related

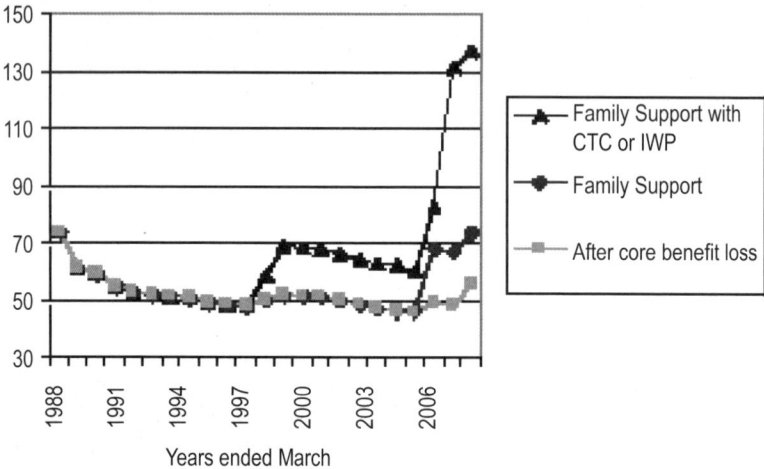

*Figure 8.6: One-child maximum per week real family assistance 1986–2008 ($2004). (Source: St John & Craig 2004)*

component of the core benefits was removed for most families: for example, a couple on a benefit with children lost $17.14 a week. Sole parents with more than one child lost $21.40. To illustrate the impact for the couple with one child family, a $20 adjustment is shown in Figure 8.6 by the third line.

Figure 8.6 makes clear that a bigger gap is opening up between the family 'in work' and those 'not in work'. For two- and three- children families the gap is less pronounced, as the In-Work Payment is set at $60 for all families of three or fewer children, but for families with four or more children the gap widens again because the In-Work Payment increases by $15 for each subsequent child. A minimum estimate of how many poor children are in these families who have been left behind can be gauged from the numbers of children recorded in families on benefits. In 2003 approximately a quarter of children under 18 (253,000 children) lived in families supported by a main social welfare benefit (Ministry of Social Development 2004). Another impact not shown in Figure 8.6 is the transformation of the third tier of supplementary assistance (the Special Benefit) into Temporary Additional Support. While the full impact of this policy is not clear, it is certain that families on benefits and low wages will be eligible for far less support than was available from a Special Benefit in 2004 (St John & Craig 2004).

## The 'In-Work Payment'

As the 2004 Working for Families package stood, families faced very long income ranges over which extra money earned would not make very much difference to their take-home pay (Nolan 2004b). For example, a family on an income of $38,000 would face a marginal tax rate of up to 74.2 per cent.

An extra $1000 earned would result in $330 tax, $300 loss of Family Support including the In-Work Payment, $100 repayment of a student loan (if there was one), and $12 in ACC levies. This leaves only $258 in the hand. In addition, other abatements could add cumulatively to the Effective Marginal Tax Rate (EMTR) such as child support payments and loss of the accommodation supplement and childcare subsidies. These high EMTRs can be assumed, a priori, to provide a significant disincentive to earn extra income.

The pre-election boost to the Working for Families package significantly raised the thresholds for abatement of Family Support and reduced the rate of abatement to 20 per cent. This is welcome in two ways. First, there is a significant boost to low-wage family income from raising the threshold, which should markedly help children in those families. Second, the EMTR problem is reduced in a way that gives a much improved work incentive. The opportunity was not taken, however, to redesign the In-Work Payment itself, and failure to include beneficiary families adds to the relative income gap that will emerge. The In-Work Payment is very generous for small families, as illustrated in Figure 8.6. Its addition was providing a significant real redistribution to families from 2006/7 but it is designed to 'reward work' rather than alleviate child poverty. The New Zealand lump-sum In-Work Payment, supposedly to 'reward not being on a benefit', has itself all the hallmarks of a welfare payment. This payment is complicated, requiring not only that neither parent be on a benefit, but also proof of hours worked. For a couple, 30 hours is required and 20 hours for a sole parent. It may prove even more difficult to administer than its predecessor, the Child Tax Credit.

Ironically the In-Work Payment makes it easier for one parent to stay home where there is a full-time breadwinner, whereas a sole parent, regardless of numbers of children, is required to work at least 20 hours a week. In reality, the In-Work Payment is structured not so much as an incentive to be in paid work, but an incentive to not receive a welfare benefit at all and a punishment for the loss of a job.

The UK also has a tax credit scheme for those in work, but it is not directly related to having children and can be received by those who do not have children. The Australians also have a different approach (St John & Craig 2004). First, they confine the EMTR problem by initially abating only part of family assistance so that a sizeable amount is essentially universal – in other words, it is received by most families except those with the highest incomes. Secondly, the tax on incomes up to $6000 is zero and part of the family assistance is abated against only the caregiver's income. Thirdly, and most significant for work incentives, the 2004 Australian budget reduced the rate at which their family tax credits abate from 30 per cent to 20 per cent, a move now followed in New Zealand as discussed above.

## Assessing income policy for children

The major focus of family assistance is currently on work incentives rather than alleviating child poverty, and this must be challenged. The In-Work Payment scheme needs to be rethought. It has many undesirable features. In particular, in terms of family assistance, it drives a large wedge between families in work and those on benefits. The presence of children is a condition of receiving it, as is the requirement that families are not on a benefit and are working the required number of hours. To that extent it is discriminatory; indeed, it has been challenged in the courts (see Child Poverty Action Group website at www.cpag.org.nz). It will be hard to administer and complex for low-income families to comply with. If there is a recession, many of the parents now receiving the In-Work Payments may lose their jobs and need to access a main benefit. This in turn could result in a sharp drop in living standards for their children. Over time, the danger is that real increases in In-Work Payment are achieved at the expense of real increases in Family Support, and the focus on reducing child poverty will be lost altogether.

Although the pre-election changes of 2005 were in the right direction, increasing the threshold for abatement of Family Support and lowering the rate at which it is withdrawn, the poorest families were ignored. As the Australians have clearly shown, improved work incentives can be achieved while still treating all children in low-income families with equal generosity. Recent studies show that poverty and poor health outcomes are clearly correlated (Shaw *et al.* 2005). Unless there is sustained intervention and the goal of reducing child poverty is given priority over providing work incentives, children unfortunate enough to be in benefit-dependent families will continue to experience poor health outcomes, higher morbidity, lower life expectancy, more school transience, and poorer educational achievement than their peers. While the improvements in family income support measures outlined in this chapter will have positive consequences for the working poor, stigmatising and excluding those on benefits cannot be in the long-term interests of society.

# 9. Health inequalities and need associated with rare diseases

John Forman

**P**ublic health priorities, whether discussed in the context of the publicly funded and provided health services or within the more specific meaning of public health as the 'science and art of preventing disease, prolonging life and promoting health through the organised efforts of society' (Acheson 1988) seem dominated in the media and public discussion, and in the policy process itself, by common conditions which affect large numbers of people and, by quick extrapolation, cost the most money.

There is little reference anywhere in current health policies to diseases and conditions that are less common than those that regularly make health priority lists or appear in health policy discussion documents, yet rare diseases that include a wide range of metabolic and neurological diseases, for example, have a substantial collective impact on the health of the whole population. In this chapter the question of health inequalities and need is approached from a layperson's perspective, focusing in particular on how rare diseases are dealt with in health policy and action plans. The conclusion is that there is systemic neglect of the health needs of a significant sector in our community, leading to significant health inequalities. Specific actions are called for to address the needs of the rare disease population.

The perspective taken is coloured by my role and interests, including my work role for the New Zealand Organisation for Rare Disorders (NZORD) (www.nzord.org.nz), and my personal interest in support groups relevant to my family involvement with rare genetic diseases – Lysosomal Diseases New Zealand (www.ldnz.org.nz) and ISMRD, the International Advocate for Glycoprotein Storage Diseases (www.ismrd.org).

Some subtle distinction needs to be made between diseases that are rare and those that are genetic; however, rare disorders are mostly genetic in origin, and most genetic diseases are rare. So despite some obvious exceptions to these rules, the phrases 'rare' and 'genetic' have substantial overlaps and commonality of interest. The particular problems they have in common are limited expertise to diagnose accurately, limited expertise in clinical care, limited investment in research, and limited establishment of policy relating to these disorders. For most of this chapter references to 'rare diseases' are made in the knowledge that genetics is the primary cause, or at least a major contributor, to most of these diseases, and that genetic knowledge and services offer the actual or potential solution to most of them (Office of Rare Diseases 2006; National Advisory Committee on Health and Disability 2003).

Important distinctions also need to be made between genetic diseases. Some genetic defects are the direct cause of certain disease states, regardless of other factors such as environment. These are generally single-gene diseases and they often have severe or life-threatening impacts on the patient, or will lead to chronic health problems. Other genetic defects may lead only to susceptibility to disease, in which case an environmental or other trigger will also be needed for the disease to manifest itself. Some susceptibility conditions can be severe and life-threatening, while others will lead to less severe chronic conditions.

To illustrate, rare diseases consist of over 9000 different diseases (National Advisory Committee on Health and Disability 2003) that occur less often than 1 in 2000 in the population, as defined in Europe (European Commission 2002), or, in the US definition, affect fewer than 200,000 Americans, which is about 1 in 1400 (Office of Rare Diseases 2006). It is widely accepted that around 8 per cent (National Organization for Rare Disorders 2006) of the entire population will be affected by a rare disease over their whole lifespan. When the effect on the immediate family is also factored in (assuming two others per household) rare diseases then impact directly or indirectly on three times 8 per cent, which is nearly 25 per cent of the population. So the individually rare is also collectively common, and thus a significant factor in the health of the whole community.

## Understanding the context of health care planning and delivery

One of the most important aspects in any discussion on rare diseases, as in many other areas of health care, is how the health care system tries to deal with them. Several significant factors are intertwined, as outlined below.

First, rare diseases do not exist in isolation, and solutions to them do not happen independently of other health services and strategies. They are tied up closely with the funding pressures, politics and priorities, the training and expertise of clinicians, and other complexities of the health system.

In addition, rare diseases have to be considered as part of a health system where there are rapidly increasing costs in most parts of the system, strong pressures to control those costs, and rapid development of health technology that is often very expensive. At the same time, there is an increasing burden of disease in the community associated with longer life expectancy, and social, environmental, and lifestyle factors that cause disease.

So at a very simple level the pressure on health care planning and delivery can be explained like this: dealing with society's disease burden solely by having a traditional model of health care expanded to provide more hospital beds and more drugs to treat disease, will inevitably lead to an increasing demand on the expensive, high-tech end of health services; in time these pressures will be unmanageable in terms of costs, the expertise needed to run them, and the sheer numbers seeking treatments, unless there are concerted efforts to develop primary interventions and community actions that prevent people from developing such severe forms of disease, and the diseases themselves from occurring so widely.

This view of the pressures in health has become well established internationally, and one of the key documents that capture some of these themes is the Ottawa Charter (World Health Organization 1986). This charter, developed in 1986, and the philosophy behind it are significant influences here in New Zealand, mainly in the form of the New Zealand Health Strategy, the Primary Health Care Strategy, the Public Health Strategy and Action Plans, and the Māori Health Strategy. The philosophy has also underpinned important discussion documents such as the National Health Committee's report on *The Social, Cultural and Economic Determinants of Health in New Zealand* (National Health Committee 1998).

Probably the greatest influence of the Ottawa Charter, from the rare-disease perspective, has been to introduce another dimension to the competition for resources that had been growing within the health services for some decades. On its own, the charter provides sound and coherent reasoning for early intervention and community action on health, and a necessary tool for reducing the demand on health services traditionally provided in hospital settings, often described as secondary and tertiary services, compared to the primary services and interventions delivered in the community.

But the charter includes a call to reorient health services 'towards health promotion and beyond its responsibility for providing clinical and curative services' (World Health Organization 1986). When this is considered along with the other themes in the charter and in the context of tight financial pressures, there just isn't enough money to go around, and competition between different parts of the health sector becomes strong.

## Competition for health resources

The rise of public health philosophy and its acceptance in health planning leads to a tension between those engaged in public health functions (organised community effort aimed at the prevention of disease and the promotion of health – not to be confused with a range of publicly funded services) and those in more traditional clinical and curative roles usually, though not always, found in secondary and tertiary services in hospital settings. In addition, the traditional clinical and curative services are competing with each other for scarce resources. No part of the health sector is getting all the resources they want. To increase their share of the health budget, they have to compete strongly with other health services that in turn feel vulnerable to the competing claims of the others.

Now add to this complicated mix the reality that if there is a shift from secondary/tertiary services, as the main thrust of health service delivery, to a primary care and public health (community action, early intervention) approach to health improvement, it is likely to take some time to bed in. Personal communications with some experienced clinicians suggest that it will take about two generations to produce real reductions in the demand for secondary/ tertiary services as a result of preventive public health approaches. It becomes clear that the availability of a range of health services will be compromised as the major shifts are made. If there is continued priority allocation of resources into primary and public health care, then waiting lists for surgery, restricted access to medicines, and delays in implementing new equipment and treatments, are the inevitable consequence, despite funding increases to the total health budget that continue to exceed the inflation rate.

This dilemma was apparent in the strategic plan for the Auckland District Health Board 2002–7, where it was stated that 'We will identify areas to make primary services more efficient, reallocating resources from low priority areas to high priority areas within primary health, and shifting resources from the secondary, tertiary and national tertiary sector into the primary services' (Auckland District Health Board 2002: 21). Later the same document states: 'and a focus on primary and ambulatory services requiring funding shifts from hospital to primary services' (Auckland District Health Board 2002: 118). The plan notes 'a substantial risk for conflict between the population health objectives of the DHB and the hospital's position as a national provider of high-cost complex services' (Auckland District Health Board 2002: 120).

Notably though, despite similar language in other District Health Board (DHB) plans of the same era, there is no specific reference to these funding shifts in the ADHB plans being developed in 2005–6, and there is now more emphasis on the maintenance of services. Personal communication with the authors of current plans suggests the need to establish more of an evidence-base for any such shifts, although the impact of submissions from interest groups have combined to mute the enthusiasm for such a course of action.

The rhetoric of shifting funds from secondary and tertiary services to primary and public health interventions has not been borne out by practice in the health sector. This is in spite of implied directives in some of the health strategy documents. Indeed it is doubtful if such an approach was ever going to succeed, given the strong protective instincts that accompany all health services and the readiness with which professionals and patient groups often respond to any suggestion of cuts to their services.

Pragmatism and political expediency should perhaps always dictate that getting new health initiatives in place is dependent on allocating new, dedicated budgets. Those advocating for improved public health initiatives may find their goals more readily achieved if their advocacy does not involve their success being dependent on a loss elsewhere.

## Impact on people with rare diseases

In short, the developments discussed above leave people with a rare disease in a continuing difficult situation, bereft of serious attention to their collective needs. The rather brief and possibly simplistic summary of health service planning and service changes given above is based largely on an existing range of services dealing with a variety of diseases that have a reasonable set of knowledge and treatment options available to them. It does not yet factor in that neither the existing nor the proposed new systems have made significant provision for the detection, diagnosis, and treatment of rare diseases.

It is true that secondary and tertiary services have been the major provider of services for these diseases, but limited knowledge of genetics and gene-function for most of the twentieth century effectively restricted medical treatment of them, with a few notable exceptions, to symptomatic and palliative care. In recent decades, as advances in genetic knowledge have greatly improved the ability to diagnose, prevent, and treat rare diseases, secondary and tertiary services are now able to do more for their management and treatment, but are also under considerable pressure, as outlined above, and consequently are considerably restricted in their ability to effectively provide treatment and care for them (National Advisory Committee on Health and Disability 2003). At the same time, the rising interest in preventative primary and public health, and advocacy associated with this interest, does not appear to have resulted in any sort of priority for those with rare diseases, nor support for the development of genetic services that are essential to their needs. Each specific technology, treatment or service for rare diseases is thus left in the invidious situation of having to be advocated for individually, in the absence of an over-arching policy that recognises their collective impacts and responds appropriately with a policy framework based on recognition of need, equity of access, social justice in resource distribution, good health economics, and reduction of disparities in health status. An example of this is the neglected state of genetic services in New Zealand. Despite a comprehensive report in 2003 from the National Health Committee (National Advisory Committee on Health and Disability 2003) on the need, the urgency, and the way to bring these services up to standard (without dealing with growth and development to meet future needs) there has been no action by the Ministry of Health or District Health Boards to implement this report.

There is a detectable concern among many advocates in the rare disease community that their needs fall into something of a black hole in the health system; and that, intentional or not, there is systematic and systemic neglect of their collective interests. Many now see the neglect as very significant, comparable perhaps to the time not so long ago when there was political blindness to the now validated impacts of social and economic determinants of health (National Health Committee 1998), or to the neglect of significant disparities in health status of Māori compared to the rest of the population, until the development of the Māori Health Strategy (Ministry of Health 2002a). Such concerns suggest that if there is a core of factors leading to health inequalities and need, then rarity should certainly be included.

The great irony is that many discussion documents on public health policy and action plans, such as that by Dahlgren and Whitehead quoted in the Ministry of Health's Public Health Action Framework (Ministry of Health 2002b), actually start with a reference to genetics. The most common reference is a diagram indicating causes of disease with the circle split in two – one half indicating our genetic makeup (including sex and hereditary factors) as a significant factor in disease risk and susceptibility, and the other half indicating environmental factors and interactions as causes of disease. The documents then move on to consider in detail the environmental aspects of disease and how strategies and action plans may limit those consequences, while the genetic factors are almost totally ignored.

## Genetic causes of disease

At this point it is useful to add some refinement to the discussion of genetic causes of disease. There are those genetic conditions (usually single-gene disorders) which will definitely lead to disease onset solely because of the genetic defect itself and regardless of environmental factors. Other genetic conditions, however, will lead to a susceptibility to disease with the actual onset of disease being subject to the influence of environmental factors. This distinction seems poorly understood in public health discussion documents, as judged by the absence of any significant reference to inheritance factors in the Public Health Action Framework. Its reference to tackling the 'root causes' of poor health refers only to environmental approaches (Ministry of Health 2002b). Moreover, this document does not recognise that population health promotion and wellness maintenance usually does nothing to stop the onset of genetically determined disease. Nor does it factor in the limited value of population health approaches for those who do not have susceptibility factors for particular diseases, or who have inherited risks that are not provided for.

There is also some irony in the fact that one of the earliest population-wide public health programmes in New Zealand was newborn screening for metabolic diseases. This programme was set up in 1969 and uses laboratory testing of blood spots from newborn babies to detect genetic or chromosome abnormalities that lead to phenylketonuria (PKU), cystic fibrosis, and five other diseases. Nearly two million New Zealand babies have been screened by this programme, and every year early detection allows treatments or interventions that deliver dramatically improved outcomes for about 30 babies who would otherwise die or be seriously affected by the condition they have.

Another significant public health programme in place for many decades is pre-natal screening for at-risk pregnancies to avoid preventable disabilities. Taking a family history in all pregnancies enables identification of pregnancies at increased risk of genetic disorders and allows for the appropriate testing to be organised in a timely fashion. Trisomies, Fragile X, anencephaly, and other disorders can be identified by amniocentesis, chorionic villie sampling (CVS) or ultrasound screening. This screening can offer choices that significantly reduce the burden on hundreds of families every year.

Neither of these important public health approaches to rare diseases gains much notice at all in public health discussions or policy. There is just one reference to the potential for incorporating genetic screening into public health in the Public Health Action Framework, and a similarly brief mention of the need to assess the impacts of the new genetics on public health. New genetics refers to developments that have resulted from gene sequencing technologies; a prominent manifestation of the new genetics is the human genome project. The existing public health screening programmes noted above are not even mentioned in the Framework (Ministry of Health 2002b).

## Reviewing the context and reaching conclusions

A summary of the discussion so far shows a health system that is going through significant changes and has significant competing pressures within it, leaving little in the way of resources to address rare diseases. Add to this a situation where public health and primary prevention approaches to health planning seem to be on the rise, yet neither acknowledge genetics or rare diseases. Now reintroduce to the argument the significant numbers of the population who are affected by rare diseases, and the significant growth in knowledge of genetic causes of disease that has arisen over the recent past.

When these factors are combined, the conclusion becomes obvious: a significant burden of disease in our population arises from rare diseases that can be diagnosed, managed, treated or prevented, thus significantly improving the health and quality of life of the affected population – yet services to deliver these outcomes are few and far between, and poorly resourced.

The consequence of this is a relatively new cohort in the population whose health needs are significantly neglected, who face increasing disparity in health status, and who are subject to inequity of access to health services. The term 'new cohort' in the population is used because, while this cohort has always existed, the ability to better understand, diagnose, treat and prevent their diseases now gives them a new status, as an underserved population with a stronger claim for the attention of health service planning .

The new power of public health philosophy, and the influence it has had in public policy, has brought many new perspectives to health care, led to developments in community action and preventative measures, and done much to begin the process of addressing health disparities and inequities. This assertion includes, as outcomes of public health philosophy in the broadest sense, the significant policy initiatives in income support for families, improvements to housing, the development of primary health organisations, workplace safety policy, and smokefree legislation, plus other major initiatives which are underway. Yet by failing to adequately address genetics and the resultant rare diseases in its literature and programmes, public health philosophy has seriously neglected a major cause of society's disease burden.

## Rare diseases are a significant public health problem

It may seem incongruous to advocate that rare diseases should be incorporated into public health philosophy and planning, when the clinicians who currently work to manage them are almost exclusively in secondary and tertiary services. Those clinicians include the genetics service itself with its experts in genetic diagnosis and explanation of inheritance and risk, plus a range of specialists in various other disciplines such as cardiology, paediatrics, metabolics, rheumatology, neurology, and others.

It may also seem incongruous when much of the debate in public health circles is so frequently competing for resources with secondary and tertiary services, and for this reason opinion leaders in public health will perhaps be less inclined to welcome the suggestion of this new agenda item and may also instinctively resist supporting expenditure on training, equipment, and other resources that would probably be substantially housed in secondary and tertiary services.

The argument presented here is based partly on a wider view of the competitive elements within the health sector. The high degree of competition between the two parts of the public health system (public health and secondary/tertiary services) is considered to be unhelpful and counter-productive. They are both essential components of a comprehensive modern health system, and they depend on each other. Talk of 'reallocating resources away from hospital to community' (Auckland District Health Board 2002), and other competitive arguments, will therefore eventually harm both parts of the sector. For example, the public health approaches of prevention and early detection and intervention will not achieve their goals if the secondary/tertiary services do not have the specialists, equipment or medicines to do the follow-up interventions or treatment indicated by the success of the public health screening or wellness promotion programmes.

Establishing rare diseases as a public health issue is important because these diseases impact on the whole population. They cannot be ignored if their collective impact is acknowledged and the total societal burden of disease is factored in. By contrast, it is relatively easy to ignore them if each disease is considered in isolation, namely in the context of a particular condition that affects just a small number of families.

A public health approach to genetics is an important part of a comprehensive approach to rare diseases. Generating genetic knowledge at a community level will help families to work with their primary health professionals to understand and manage their risk of genetic disease, through public awareness, screening, and diagnosis. It is important to note, however, that the expertise of specialists in genetic services and other secondary/tertiary services will often be needed to confirm the diagnosis and manage the prevention and treatment strategies.

In this part of the discussion, it is also worth noting that in both the United States and the European Union, public policy has recognised rare diseases as a significant public health problem (European Commission 2002), requiring specific policies and resources to address them.

# What is achievable now?

This section offers some specific examples that demonstrate the beneficial health outcomes that are achievable from validated interventions or specific services for rare diseases.

## Newborn metabolic screening can be expanded

Advances in technology can add more than 25 severe but treatable disorders to newborn metabolic screening. These include amino acid disorders, fatty acid oxidation disorders, and organic acid disorders, with much improved outcomes if detected early for up to ten babies each year (Ministry of Health 2005).

## Newborn hearing screening is now possible

A simple but reliable test could identify about 170 cases of permanent congenital hearing loss each year, and allow early intervention with speech and learning strategies during the critical first years (Ministry of Health 2006a).

## Inherited cardiac diseases can be identified in at risk families

Sudden cardiac deaths in otherwise healthy people can be a sign of inherited cardiac arrhythmias that can be tested for and treated in relatives, saving up to 30 or 40 lives a year (Cardiac Inherited Diseases Group 2005).

## Folate fortification of food can prevent neural tube defect

An estimated reduction of around 20 fatal or seriously disabling neural tube defects per year can be achieved by adding the dietary supplement folic acid to food supplies (New Zealand Food Safety Authority/Ministry of Health 2004).

## Pre-natal screening for foetal aneuploidy can be significantly improved

Better screening methods can give more accurate and reliable tests for several preventable conditions that are fatal or cause significant disability, greatly reducing procedure-related foetal loss among women screened (Stone & Austin 2006).

Pre-implantation genetic diagnosis (PGD) for prevention of inherited diseases would also have been on this list, had not the government, in December 2005, announced funding for PGD for couples at risk. This will provide government funding to approximately 50 couples per year who are at known risk of a serious inherited disease in any pregnancy. Of the items listed above, a universal newborn hearing screening was the subject of commitments during the 2005 election campaign, with funding confirmed in the 2006 budget, and at the time of writing work is underway to expand newborn metabolic screening.

If all these examples were implemented, along with the National Health Committee's recommended improvements to genetic services, there would be significant improvements to health outcomes for many hundreds of New Zealand families every year. Indicative totals are the avoidance of significant morbidity and mortality for about 350 families each year.

## What are the barriers to progress?

There are two major impediments to progress in addressing the health needs of those affected by rare diseases. The first is the absence of a comprehensive policy to deal with them. The second is fragmented responsibility for the component parts.

The recent history of success with PGD policy and service delivery, and progress with universal newborn hearing screening, show quite clearly that at present each aspect of rare diseases needs to be advocated for in isolation. There is no over-arching policy that draws together the themes and connections. As a consequence much of the work needed to progress them is reliant on political support (and pressure) for the specific initiatives.

Within the Ministry of Health, the Clinical Services Directorate is responsible for ante-natal and pre-natal services, the Disability Service Directorate is responsible for the ongoing support costs for the patient and their family, the Sector Policy Directorate is responsible for developments relating to innovations and ethics of new technologies, and the Public Health Directorate is responsible for national screening programmes (Ministry of Health 2006b). DHB New Zealand has the task of implementing the genetic services review, and the New Zealand Food Safety Authority (NZFSA) is responsible for decisions about food fortification with supplements. With such fragmented responsibilities and the absence of a policy to focus the work, it is perhaps inevitable that the needs of those with rare diseases are poorly met and the health inequalities associated with them remain substantially unaddressed.

Given the large number of groups with a stake in meeting the health care needs of people with rare diseases, some coordination is urgently needed and it is suggested that the Sector Policy Directorate should have responsibility for implementation work on setting up a new policy to provide for those with rare diseases – a key part of which would be the inclusion of comprehensive genetic services. That directorate should also be given the task of coordinating the work of other directorates, the NZFSA and the DHBs to provide comprehensive services to meet the needs of the rare disease community.

## What should the policy contain?

A coherent approach to the policy issue could reflect that of a position paper on the needs of rare diseases, recently adopted by the International Genetic Alliance. NZORD is a participant in this Alliance. The position paper sets out four key principles (New Zealand Organisation for Rare Disorders 2007):

1. Rare diseases are a significant public health issue. They affect around 8 per cent of the population and when the immediate family is factored in, rare diseases impact on nearly 25 per cent of the population.

- In many countries 8 per cent is equivalent to the size of significant minority populations. Just as leaving the health needs of such a population unmet would be unacceptable and discriminatory, so is the neglect of equivalent populations affected by rare diseases.

2. Health care and treatment for rare diseases is a human rights issue. Non-discrimination, justice, and equity of access to health care, all require that specific policies are put in place to address the needs of people affected by rare diseases.

   - Responses such as prioritisation and the need to ration resources, as reasons for lesser attention to rare diseases in health research, planning and service delivery, are not ethically sustainable arguments.

3. A comprehensive approach to rare diseases is needed, including education, research, prevention, diagnosis, care, and treatment.

   - Services and support for patients and families need to be holistic and integrated to provide for the many health, disability and social issues often associated with them.

4. Quality information, informed consent, and autonomous decision-making are critical for upholding the rights and the protection of patients and their families in all aspects of treatment, research, and prevention.

   - Combining genetic knowledge with newborn screening, pre-natal screening, and other detection methods to identify risk should be actively pursued to give parents choice about prevention, but this must be balanced with careful attention to informed consent and autonomous decision-making.

A number of specific implementation issues flow from these principles, including the importance of integration of the public health approach with clinical service delivery. Indeed, by adopting such an approach our government and health services would be taking a timely step in addressing the needs of a significant section of our population who do not feature as prominently as they should on the radar screens of most parts of the health sector.

Public health approaches cover a broad spectrum of actions, actual and potential, but for an area of health that enjoys robust discussion and many thoughtful contributions, public health policy has been surprisingly slow to note the significance of genetics and the importance of rare diseases as part of its mandate.

# Part Three
## Intervention Strategies

# 10. Why are we weighting? Equity considerations in primary health care resource allocation formulas

Peter Crampton and Jon Foley

This chapter examines the construction of New Zealand's primary health care funding formulas. These funding formulas have major health implications as they provide the public funding life-blood that keeps the primary health care system running. The aim of the chapter is to explore the equity implications of using different weighting variables in funding formulas. In particular the chapter examines the relative merits of socio-demographic variables (such as socio-economic deprivation and ethnicity) and health variables (such as measures of morbidity and mortality).

The chapter starts with a brief overview of New Zealand's experience with funding formulas and the ethics that underlie these formulas. This is followed by a description of, and the rationale for, the set of primary health care funding formulas current in 2006. Alternative approaches to risk adjustment are then described. The final section of the chapter outlines the pros and cons of different approaches New Zealand could adopt for constructing funding formulas.

Health system funding mechanisms can be grouped into broad categories: private out-of-pocket expenditure, private health insurance, social health insurance, and state funding of health services. Many wealthy countries, including New Zealand, aim to ensure equitable access to health care using funding systems that are based, partly or largely, on need for health services and not willingness-to-pay (van Doorslaer *et al.* 2005). This chapter is concerned with the mechanisms used in New Zealand to distribute state funds to primary health care services on the basis of population need. The equity implications of different funding mechanisms are described elsewhere (for example, Starfield 1998).

About 80 per cent of total health care resources come from government sources – in real terms Vote Health expenditure alone amounted to more than eight billion dollars for the 2003/4 financial year (Ministry of Health 2005). These government funds cascade through the health system and are dispersed to a large extent on the basis of particular formulas (Figure 10.1). The district health board funding formula allocates public funds to the 21 district health boards based largely on the number of people within each board's region. These per-head allowances are then adjusted so that young people and older people receive a greater per-capita allowance (consistent with their greater need for health services), as do those living in socio-economically deprived areas,[1] and

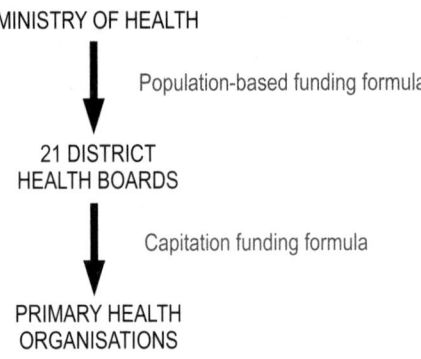

*Figure 10.1: The funding cascade*

Māori and Pacific populations. Adjustments are also made for district health boards with rural populations and for those with high numbers of overseas visitors. A proportion of each regional allocation is passed on to primary health organisations using four related funding formulas: the First-Contact formula, the Services to Improve Access formula, the Health Promotion funding formula, and the Care Plus formula (Hefford *et al*. 2005). These four formulas are described in more detail later in the chapter.

Formulas have been a dominant feature of health system funding in this country since the 1980s. The next section describes the political and technical origins of our funding formulas, including the social and policy objectives that they aim to achieve.

## Equity in health care resource allocation
The ethical foundation for New Zealand's now well-established approach to health care funding was laid down by the 1938 Social Security Act. Embedded in this approach were utilitarian principles that placed value on promoting overall population health gain – the greatest good for the greatest number – as reflected in the provision, in 1938, of universal tax-financed primary and secondary medical care, and prescriptions, free of charge to the patient (Oliver 1988: 25). Alongside these utilitarian principles, and distinct from them, was a commitment to distributive justice – a commitment to fairness in resource allocation (Beauchamp & Childress 1989: 261) – which was reflected in the desire to assist those most in need and, implicitly, to reduce health inequalities. This aim was given expression in the needs-based approach to medical benefits (care would be provided by the state according to medical needs of individuals without regard to their ability to pay (Royal Commission of Inquiry on Social Security in New Zealand 1972: 394)), and the introduction of means-tested benefits for those unable to earn for themselves (Oliver 1988: 25).

The concept of medical need has spawned a rich discussion in the economics literature. A useful definition of need is that a person (or population) has a need where there is the capacity to benefit from health care (Birch & Chambers 1993). As might be expected, there is a range of approaches to translating the concept of need, defined as capacity to benefit, into something more measurable.

At a population level, need for health care resources is related most fundamentally to population size, as well as the age and sex structure of a population. Over and above population numbers and age, it is not possible to encapsulate need for health care using any single population characteristic. Hence the measurement of need frequently focuses on summary health measures, such as the mortality experience of a population, or when such data are not available or are considered to be unsuitable, on socio-economic measures. Both these approaches have been used for needs-based resource allocation for health services in the United Kingdom, Canada, and in New Zealand. For example, standardised mortality ratios[2] were first introduced into a formula for resource allocation for hospital services in the United Kingdom in 1977 (Eyles et al. 1991).

The 1980 report of the Advisory Committee on Hospital Board Funding, referred to as the 'Blue Book' (Advisory Committee on Hospital Board Funding 1980), was a watershed in the history of resource allocation in New Zealand. Prior to this, little effort had been made to systematically address population needs-based funding of health services in New Zealand. The 'Blue Book' was the first such attempt.[3] Population needs-based funding of hospital and related services was subsequently introduced in New Zealand in 1983 (Advisory Committee on Hospital Board Funding 1986), and has been the cornerstone of health service funding ever since, despite almost continuous restructuring of the health system.

A form of population-based funding, known as capitation funding, has been used to varying extents in primary health care for the past 60 years. Capitation funding means per head funding of general practitioner (GP) patients, whereby monthly government payments are made to practices according to the number of patients on their books, rather than how many times those patients actually visit. The advantages of capitation funding include the ability to distribute funding more equitably in a planned way; the incentive to care for enrolled populations on a longitudinal basis rather than per procedure or per visit; the ability to target resources to practices serving high needs enrollees; and, promotion of a team approach because funding is not tied to the GP providing services directly to every patient (Crampton et al. 2002).

The principles of capitation funding were first introduced into the primary health care sector in the 1940s (Crampton et al. 2002; Medical Services Committee 1948), but remained out of favour amongst GPs and were little used prior to National's health reforms in 1993. Up until then most GPs were funded on a fee-for-service basis – that is, they claimed a government subsidy each time a patient visited. Moves to capitation funding of individual general practices accelerated during the 1990s.

The Labour government's Primary Health Care Strategy (King 2001), released in 2001, added new impetus to the trend towards capitation funding of primary health care services by introducing 'needs-based funding for population care' to (partly) replace fee-for-service funding approaches.

## Existing primary health care funding formulas

At the time of writing (late 2005), PHO funding was allocated on a per capita basis using a cluster of related formulas (Hefford *et al.* 2005). Figure 10. 2 provides an overview of the different formulas.

| Formula Name | Services Funded | Key Variables | Other Features |
|---|---|---|---|
| First Contact (Access) | Core GP and nursing services offered in primary care practices | Age, gender, High User Health Card | PHO or practice must have 50 per cent of enrollees Māori, Pacific or NZDep 9/10 decile or be in a district with 50 per cent of residents with these characteristics |
| First Contact (Interim) | Core GP and nursing services offered in primary care practices | Age, gender, Community Services Card, High User Health Card | <25 and >64 funded using rates that are the same or similar to Access |
| Services to Improve Access | Locally-determined outreach and extension services designed to improve access for high need populations | Age, gender, NZDep, ethnicity | Funding based on the number of enrollees who are Māori, Pacific or NZDep 9/10 decile |
| Health Promotion | Population-based health promotion services | NZDep, ethnicity | Coordinated with other public health initiatives |
| Care Plus | Enhanced services for the most medically complex enrollees | Age, gender, NZDep, ethnicity | Comprises on average 5 per cent PHO enrollees; funding capped based on projected caseload |
| Management Services | Management of PHO services | Size of the enrolled population | 3 sets of rates based on size of the PHO; rates reflect economies of scale |

*Figure 10.2: Existing primary health care funding formulas (2005)*

The First Contact formulas were developed using data on GP claims for general medical services from the 1998/9 year (Sutton 2000). In addition, where GP claiming data were not available (in the case of those who were not eligible for government subsidies), data from a survey of practice activity in the mid-1990s were used (Gribben 1996). These two data sources, when combined, reflected utilisation of GP services by age, gender, and Community Services Card (CSC) status (where eligibility for a CSC is tied to family income). No comparable data were available by ethnicity or deprivation status; however, based on analysis of the New Zealand Health Survey (Scott *et al*. 2003), it was estimated that Māori and Pacific populations consulted their GP at about the same rate as the rest of the population, despite having poorer health status.

The Primary Health Care Strategy, launched in 2000, set out a 10-year strategy for fundamental improvements to primary health care access, delivery, and quality. Because one of the principal aims of the strategy was reducing health inequalities, the Ministry of Health recommended that additional resources be directed at those who have historically missed out on care (defined as Māori, Pacific, and those residing in deprivation decile 9 and 10 areas). Using deprivation and ethnicity in any First Contact formula was problematic for two reasons. First, there was not much evidence related to GP use by ethnicity and deprivation, and what evidence did exist indicated that these groups seek care at rates similar to the rest of the population despite being sicker (HURA Research Alliance *et al*. 2006; Scott *et al*. 2003). Hence, even if data could be obtained to support an allocation by ethnicity and deprivation, the resulting formula would cement in place historical inequities and contravene the aim of the strategy.

Assuming that GP utilisation data were available by ethnicity and deprivation, one could apply a weighting to reflect the additional need experienced by Māori and Pacific populations. However, this assumes that there is information on the 'optimal' level of GP services that high needs populations require. There is no evidence that suggests what this level should be. Moreover, it is not clear that funding additional GP care is the most effective way of improving access for high needs populations. Based on the work of community clinics such as those affiliated with Health Care Aotearoa[4] (Crampton *et al*. 2001), alternative approaches such as community health workers or marae-based clinics were thought to be more effective ways of reaching these people.

This line of thinking led to the development of the Services to Improve Access (SIA) formula. Using the community health worker approach as a model, Ministry of Health analysts estimated the amount of funding required to support a community health worker to provide outreach services to a manageable number of high needs primary care users. The level of funding was then translated into formula weightings. SIA funding for Māori or Pacific enrollees residing in the most deprived areas was based on 40 per cent of the Access First Contact amount by age and gender; Māori or Pacific enrollees in less deprived areas received a 20 per cent weighting; Pākehā enrollees in deprived areas also drew a 20 per cent weighting, and the rest were not funded for SIA.

Under the Health Promotion formula, all populations draw some level of funding (a uniform base level of $2 per enrollee); however, this base amount is increased by the SIA weightings for Māori, Pacific, and people living in deprived areas. The logic for the differences between the SIA and Health Promotion is that all enrollees can benefit from population-based health promotion programmes, whereas only certain populations require improved access. PHOs receive the same level of SIA and Health Promotion funding regardless of whether they are Access (serving primarily high needs) or Interim (serving average and well-off populations).

The Care Plus funding formula was based on a 60,000-person sample of patients from three sets of practices where there was thought to be accurate coding of chronic diseases. From this sample, analysts determined the expected number of people who were high users or had one or more chronic diseases. Despite the fact that Māori, Pacific, and more deprived people are known to suffer higher rates of morbidity and premature death due to chronic diseases, the sample population included fewer of them than their proportion in the sample population. This suggested that people with high needs either were not seeking care at the same rate or, once enrolled, were not being identified as having certain chronic diseases. Hence, the SIA weightings were applied to the Care Plus formula so as not to perpetuate historical inequities.

## Risk rating using health information

Risk rating refers to the process of adjusting payments so that funding takes account of the need for health services in a fair way. The selection of variables to use in capitation formulas is influenced by a number of factors. To a certain extent, capitation formulas in New Zealand have been designed to reflect known patterns of use or resource consumption. In practice, however, these formulas also are attempting to provide incentives for health planners and practitioners to achieve societal goals (for example, addressing unmet need) and efficiency. In a survey of capitation formulas across 20 developed countries, Rice and Smith (2001: 91) concluded:

> Essentially, a capitation system seeks to answer the question as to how – given that health care expenditure is to be constrained – the limited resources available should be distributed among health care plans in accordance with society's equity and efficiency objectives. The purpose of risk-adjusted capitation is to ensure that plans will receive the same level of funding for people in equal need of health care, regardless of extraneous circumstances such as residence and level of income.

Most capitation formulas currently used by health service organisations, whether in private insurance markets or public sector programmes, are based on demographic factors (generally age and sex) or demographic factors plus socio-economic factors (deprivation or income-based measures). Researchers and planners have acknowledged that these factors are only proxies for health need. When used to allocate funding across large, representative populations, these proxies may accurately reflect patterns of resource consumption or health need. However, for smaller population groups or where the population is not representative, they are not necessarily accurate (Majeed *et al*. 2001).

Many studies have demonstrated that age- or gender-based capitation formulas better reflect health needs when measures of morbidity and mortality are included (Shen & Ellis 2002). From a statistical standpoint, adding more variables will always add to the explanatory power, so consideration has to be given to the marginal cost (in terms of data collection, transparency, ease of use) of adding more variables together with the relative power of new variables in explaining health care costs.

In their survey of developed countries (not including the US) regarding the variables used in capitation formulas, Rice and Smith classified variables based on whether the underlying data used to develop the formulas were at an individual level or at a 'plan' level (meaning they were aggregated data from sources such as the census). Of the 20 countries they surveyed in 2000, none used mortality as a variable in capitation formulas at an individual level; Finland and the Netherlands used disability status at an individual level; Sweden used previous inpatient diagnosis at an individual level; Australia (New South Wales), Belgium, England, Italy, Northern Ireland, Scotland, and Norway used mortality at a plan level; and England was the only country to use morbidity at a plan level. In comparison, the core primary care capitation formulas (First Contact) used in New Zealand were developed primarily on data (such as age and gender) collected at an individual level.

## Morbidity-based risk adjustment

Rice and Smith assessed the various types of variables used in funding formulas: age/sex, ethnicity, employment/disability status, geographical location, mortality, morbidity, and other social factors. While many of the non-morbidity types of variables are more readily available, they concluded that morbidity 'is the individual characteristic most closely related to health care needs, and can be an important risk adjustment variable in systems that seek to avoid cream skimming'[5] (Rice & Smith 2001: 104). However, historically, morbidity data have not been used often outside the US for risk rating, in part because they are not collected and analysed routinely and consistently.

In the US, most state Medicaid Programs (state-managed health insurance for the poor and disabled) operate capitation programmes covering all or a portion of people eligible for Medicaid (Holohan *et al*. 1999). A survey of these programmes by the Urban Institute in 1999 showed that most used a variety of demographic variables to adjust for risk. Where health status measures were used, they tended to be fairly crude (for example, by single condition such as pregnancy or HIV/AIDs). However, a handful of states (Colorado, Maryland, Michigan, Minnesota, and Washington) reported that they were implementing or considering more sophisticated risk adjustment systems that rely on morbidity data. Since this survey was conducted, more states have ventured into morbidity-based risk capitation systems.

The US Medicare Program (federal health insurance for the elderly and disabled) has historically paid health providers on a fee-for-service basis. However, since the late 1990s, some Medicare managed care programmes have been in operation. Initially, Medicare employed a model known as the Principal Inpatient Diagnostic Cost Group (PIPDCG) to pay managed care providers. This model is based on demographic factors, disability status, and one of approximately 30 diagnostic categories based on the principal diagnosis for hospital admissions in the past year. The use of hospital admission data was seen as an interim measure, adopted for purely practical purposes, that would be overtaken by more sophisticated methodologies reliant on diagnoses from hospital and non-hospital settings (Pope *et al*. 2000).

From the late 1980s, several case-mix risk-adjustment mechanisms have emerged using morbidity data from hospital and non-hospital settings. These primarily have been used in the US in the managed care market to pay for a comprehensive range of services. The oldest of these is the Adjusted Clinical Group (ACG) system developed at Johns Hopkins University (Weiner *et al*. 1992). This system is used in several states (California, Maryland, Minnesota, Oregon, and Washington) to allocate resources for Medicaid beneficiaries. A number of countries (Sweden, Germany, Spain, and Canada) have used the ACG system to allocate resources or analyse resource use. The system is based on the notion that a person's disease burden is best described using a cluster of conditions rather than a single condition. Although the ACG coding system is derived from codes commonly used in primary care, hospital outpatient, and hospital inpatient systems across the US, it can also be adapted to other countries where different coding systems are used. According to its developers, the person-focused nature of the ACG system, where the emphasis is on an individual's disease burden rather than a particular procedure, distinguishes it from other systems (Weiner & Abrams 2001). Also unlike other systems, it classifies all persons into diagnostic groups, not just those with severe or disabling conditions.

Researchers at Boston University have developed a system known as Diagnostic Cost Groups (DxCG) (Zhao *et al*. 2002). Similar to the ACG system, the DxCG system is based on groups of conditions known as 'condition categories', which are in turn based on standard codes used in inpatient and out-of-hospital settings. A person can be placed in more than one condition category, but is classified into a single category when population profiles are created. DxCG methods also use pharmacy data to further refine the classification of individual disease burden. The DxCG system is used in 245 payment systems (private and public) including the US Medicare Program.

A third major risk-rating system, known as the Chronic Illness and Disability Payment System (CDPS) (Kronick *et al*. 2000), was developed at the University of California, San Diego. Like the ACG and DxCG systems, the CDPS relies on clusters of diagnoses to classify individuals' disease burdens. As the name suggests, CDPS is particularly adept at classifying persons with chronic conditions and excludes low cost diagnoses and ill-defined diagnoses that often complicate classification. The CDPS is designed specifically for the Medicaid market, where enrollees have a disproportionate number of disabling and chronic conditions. This system is used in a number of state Medicaid programmes, including Delaware, Michigan, Washington, and Utah.

Since Rice and Smith conducted their survey, two of the surveyed countries have moved to forms of morbidity-based risk rating. In 2002 the Netherlands adopted a risk-rating system based on certain drugs prescribed in an outpatient setting (known as Pharmacy-based Costs Groups (PCGs)) (van den Ven *et al.* 2004). The list of drugs used in this classification system is limited to those prescribed for 13 conditions where the linkage between the condition and the prescribed drug is unambiguous and the likelihood of perverse incentives and moral hazard is limited.[6]

Germany, which experienced problems with risk selection in its risk-rating system based on age, sex, income, and incapacity to work, has added a high-risk pool for those people with certain chronic diseases (Busse 2004). The Disease Management Programs (DMPs) have been introduced as a means of ensuring that sickness funds (essentially, health plans) are fairly compensated for increased risk, but are also designed to stimulate improvements in quality of care through adoption of evidence-based standards and closer integration of care in a health system which has historically been rigidly segmented.

The following figure provides a comparison of the overall ability of the formulas to explain variation in cost under varying circumstances.

The first observation is that the R squared values are low; at best, these models explain 18 per cent of the variation in health care cost. Second, all of the morbidity-based models have greater predictive power than the age/sex model

| Model | Persons with disability* | Aid to Families with Dependent Children (adults) | Aid to Families with Dependent Children (children) | General population (all ages) |
|---|---|---|---|---|
| CDPS | 0.183 | 0.083 | 0.041 | n/a |
| HCC/DCG | 0.143 | 0.080 | 0.031 | 0.109** |
| ACG | 0.098 | 0.069 | 0.031 | 0.081** |
| PCG | n/a | n/a | n/a | 0.118*** |
| Prior year | n/a | n/a | n/a | 0.081 |
| Age/sex | n/a | n/a | n/a | 0.020 |

*Figure 10.3: Predicted accuracy of different risk adjustment methods in explaining variation in cost (R squared values).[7] * See Kronick (2000) ** See Shen and Ellis (2002) *** See van den Ven et al (2004)*

(by 4:1 or 5:1); however, the model based on prior year cost is as good as the ACG model in explaining costs for the privately insured sample. Third, the models are better at explaining costs for the most needy groups (disabled) and less accurate at explaining the costs for less complicated groups (children).

### Mortality-based risk adjustment

Mortality data are used by some countries to allocate resources across large population groups; however, they are not used to allocate resources for smaller groups. There are approximately 28,000 deaths in New Zealand each year. When carved up among the 80 PHOs (median population of 21,000), there will be only an average of 88 deaths per PHO per quarter and unstable rates are likely. Moreover, mortality may not have more predictive power than other variables: a study in Quebec showed that the addition of a socio-economic variable to an age/gender adjusted capitation formula had more explanatory power than the addition of a mortality variable (Hutchison *et al*. 2000).

If district or regional mortality statistics were used in PHO formulas, this would mask the differences between PHOs. This would be particularly profound for PHOs whose enrolled population is significantly different from the district or regional population.

## Strengths and weaknesses of different risk-adjustment mechanisms

The primary health care funding formulas currently in use all use socio-demographic variables as proxy measures of need. These variables have the huge benefit of being readily available and relatively cheap to collect.

The ethnicity variable, however, has proved to be vulnerable to political challenges. In the lead-up to the 2005 general election, the question arose in political and public debates as to why both socio-economic factors (deprivation) and ethnicity factors (Māori and Pacific) were included in the primary health care funding formulas – the so-called 'race-based funding' debate. Ostensibly, the answer to this question is straightforward enough, namely that epidemiological evidence strongly points to the fact that Māori health status is not the result of poverty alone. The fact is that even when socio-economic deprivation is taken into account, Māori health status is poorer than non-Māori health status (Blakely *et al*. 2002; Ministry of Health and University of Otago 2006; Pearce *et al*. 1993; Salmond & Crampton 2000). Therefore, at a population level, Māori ethnicity is associated with need for health services over and above need associated with socio-economic deprivation. This in turn provides the rationale for having both deprivation and ethnicity in the funding allocation process: they are both needs factors that have to be taken into account.

But the 'race-based funding' debate raised a more fundamental issue: should we be using demographic factors as proxies for need in our funding formulas? Are there more accurate and fairer ways of measuring need? Is the use of ethnicity in funding formulas so socially divisive as to overcome its justification on epidemiologic grounds? Prime Minister Helen Clark described the use of Māori ethnicity in funding formulas as 'lazy' (Campbell 2005). In part, the problem with needs-based resource allocation is a technical one; it is necessary to have practical measures of need that can be used in funding formulas. However, given the level of debate around ethnicity in the formulas (which became part of a government-wide review of allocation based on ethnicity in government programmes), the choice of variables in funding formulas is as much political as it is technical. Perhaps there are better approaches than the use of demographic proxies. Some of the pros and cons associated with the use of health-based measures are discussed below.

Morbidity-based capitation formulas have been developed to provide a means for more accurately predicting or explaining health need. In the context of capitation payment systems, the use of morbidity-based formulas helps overcome adverse selection, where health plans or providers avoid enrolling less well individuals because of the cost of care. In addition to their use in capitation payment systems, Majeed *et al.* (2001) described their value in three specific areas: refining performance management rating systems such that they reflect case-mix, measuring the health of populations, and planning resource use. The following figure provides a summary of the advantages and disadvantages of using morbidity-based systems.

| Potential Advantages | Potential Disadvantages |
| --- | --- |
| Reduces risk of adverse selection | Adds to administrative complexity and may increase administrative costs |
| Provides information useful for planning and monitoring health services | Leaves a large proportion of differences in spending unexplained |
| May lead to fairer methods of resource allocation | Not adequate in explaining expenditure associated with high cost disorders |
| Provides case-mix adjusted measures of performance | May encourage the further fragmentation of health systems and a loss of population focus |
| Provides measures of the health status of primary care populations | Current approaches do not use information on patients' social and cultural circumstances, which could be important predictors of use of health services |
| Encourages providers to ensure that clinical records are complete and accurate | Different methods of risk adjustment may give very different results |
| Should help improve the process of clinical governance | |

*Figure 10.4: Advantages and disadvantages of morbidity-based risk adjustment. (Source: Majeed et al. 2001: 608)*

Though morbidity-based risk-rating systems have been in existence for 20 years, they are only just beginning to be used widely by health systems. As a result, it is still somewhat early to comment on all of the issues that they present. Still, they hold promise in terms of more accurately targeting resources.

Rice and Smith (2001: 94) offer six reasons for the slow uptake of such systems. First, relevant data are often in short supply; second, research evidence on appropriate needs factors is often sparse, dated or ambiguous in its implications; third, there is great difficulty in establishing the extent to which a particular needs factor is independent of other needs factors (that is, in handling covariances between needs factors); fourth, it is difficult to disentangle legitimate needs factors from other policy and supply influences on utilisation; fifth, it is often difficult to identify the health care costs associated with a proven needs factor; and, finally, the recipients of devolved budgets often feel they have a clear idea about which needs factors will favour their plan, and so will seek to influence the choice of needs factors through the political process.

Most morbidity-based systems rely on robust coding of primary health care events. In New Zealand, though the Read coding system is predominant, there is no uniform coding system and the version of the Read system currently in use in New Zealand is no longer supported internationally. Also, it is significant that primary care diagnostic data are not used in any payment systems at present. International experience suggests that where clinical data are not used for a payment purpose (and therefore subject to routine audit), the quality and consistency of the recording is suspect.

There is a huge difference between the current situation, where few primary care events are recorded universally, and the state of affairs in other countries (mainly the US) where morbidity-based systems rely on a very high level of accurate coding of primary care events. There would need to be a significant culture change among New Zealand GPs before such systems could be incorporated into their daily routines. The costs of this change, in terms of reconfiguring the practice's management system and opportunity cost (alternative use of resources) to general practice care could be considerable.

It is important to recall that all of the morbidity-based systems described in this chapter have been designed to allocate resources for a comprehensive range of health services, whereas the review of ethnicity in the PHO formulas is concerned with allocating approximately 10 per cent of primary care capitation payments. The financial risk in primary care is much less than that for specialty and hospital care, and the fact that only a very small portion of primary care services are being considered lessens the risk even further.

Most risk-adjustment systems are designed to allocate future resources, and this allocation is based in large part on past utilisation. Where certain groups have under-utilised services in the past relative to their health need, formulas based on past use will cement in place current funding inequalities. It is largely for this reason that ethnicity was not proposed for use in the PHO First Contact formulas: the available evidence suggested that Māori enrollees consulted their GPs as often or slightly less often than their Pākehā counterparts after taking health status into account (in other words, Māori utilisation of services was low in relation to need) (Scott *et al.* 2003).

## Conclusion

New Zealand has adopted a set of primary health care capitation formulas based on demographic variables that are proxies for health care needs. These demographic variables have the advantage of being readily available and relatively cheap to obtain. There is scope for introducing morbidity variables into the formulas, but not before considerable technical and practical hurdles have been overcome. The payoff from the investment required to implement morbidity-based formulas would need to exceed the mere allocation of a portion of primary care funding. For example, if the purpose of the morbidity-based formulas was extended to include resource planning across primary and secondary care or to measure system efficiency and productivity, the benefits may justify the costs. Still, it is by no means certain that morbidity-based formulas for primary health care would result in fairer resource allocation than the demographic-based formulas they would be replacing.

The single greatest challenge is to include in formulas variables aimed at explicitly reducing health inequalities (rather than perpetuating historical funding patterns). Rice and Smith noted that policy-makers in most of the countries they reviewed emphasise the importance of addressing health inequalities; however, almost none of them matched this rhetoric with concrete steps. They concluded: 'few practical attempts have been made so far to adjust capitation payments in order to address inequalities in health (an exception is the modest adjustment made for minority ethnic groups in the New Zealand Population Based Funding Formula)... In practice, seeking to offer equal access to health care to those in equal need has hitherto been the equity objective – either explicit or implicit – underlying almost all schemes' (Rice & Smith 2001: 87).

New Zealand has made some progress towards reducing health inequalities with the introduction of the SIA formula. Considerably more work is required to strengthen the capacity of the funding formulas to reduce inequalities. Both demographic and health status variables should be explored to this end.

# 11. The promise of primary health care

Julia Carr and Lee Tan

In the light of international evidence that demonstrates the contribution of effective primary health care in reducing disparities in health (Bunker *et al*. 1994; Starfield 1994; Shi 1997; Lantz *et al*. 1998; Shi *et al*. 1999), New Zealand has embraced primary health care as a key mechanism to address socio-economic and ethnic inequalities in this arena. Implicit in this approach is support for a dynamic movement for change from both the community and the health sector, intersectoral action to address population health issues, and more equitable distribution of health resources. This chapter outlines some of the background to the Primary Health Care Strategy and explores early implementation in terms of likely impacts on socio-economic and ethnic inequalities.

In 2000, the New Zealand government launched the country's first Primary Health Care (PHC) strategy and announced significant additional investment in primary health care. In the policy lead-up and in the strategy itself, a broad approach to improving health and reducing inequalities was signalled, consistent with primary health care as articulated in the Declaration of Alma-Ata, 1978 (World Health Organization 1978). The PHC strategy emphasises accessible primary care services, including general practice, and develops the concept of Primary Health Organisations to enable a population health focus, health promotion, and community participation.

A National Health Committee (NHC) publication in 1998 exploring the social, cultural, and economic determinants of health in New Zealand (National Advisory Committee on Health and Disability 1998) was influential in creating a climate of urgency to address inequalities in health status between population groups in New Zealand. As well as emphasising the importance of structural determinants of health, this work summarised international evidence for effective interventions, including primary health care, and provided options for the development of new policy responses.

A second National Health Committee report followed, exploring the effectiveness of primary health care, including population health approaches for reducing inequalities (National Health Committee 2000). This report was particularly influential in documenting the strength of evidence around cost barriers to health care and the differential impact on high needs populations.

As a result of the identification of these issues, the committee recommended that the government adopt a broad approach to reducing inequalities: working with communities and individuals to improve their health; addressing the broader social, cultural, economic determinants of health; allocating public funding based on the need of the population served; minimising access barriers, particularly cost and cultural barriers; and ensuring effective interventions are delivered to people most likely to benefit. Several other influential publications reinforced both the extent of health inequalities in New Zealand and the value of a systematic response (Te Puni Kōkiri 1998; Ministry of Health 1999; Howden-Chapman, Tobias, *et al*. 2000; King 2000).

The primary care sector in the late 1990s was a mix of many different service and funding models. These included community-owned primary care services, Māori providers, Pacific providers, single general practice businesses, and general practices 'organised' into Independent Practitioner Associations (IPAs). Most community-owned, Māori, and Pacific primary care services were not-for-profit entities, with salaried health professionals operating in a broad team approach to service delivery. Most general practice within the IPAs was based on a fee-for-service, GP-owned commercial model with the IPA providing a political voice and corporate services. Contracting for primary health care had become widely accepted, but little impact on inequalities was evident, and population level indicators such as ambulatory-sensitive hospitalisations were trending upward.[1] While the not-for-profit sector had developed many 'niche' services with low fees, there was a considerable cost barrier for most people wanting to access primary care services. In this way New Zealand was unusual, having free access to secondary care but a significant barrier to primary care.

The Primary Health Care Strategy, launched in 2001, provided a strong framework for intervention (King 2001). In essence, the strategy reorganises primary care providers into loose coalitions, with joint governance, population-based funding, and a responsibility for population health outcomes as well as clinical service delivery. Primary Health Organisations (PHOs) are formed by any number of providers of general practice and other primary health care, social service providers, and community groups. The enrolled population is based on those enrolled with participating general practices. Individuals are encouraged to enrol with one general practice or primary care service, but can use others as a casual patient, paying higher fees.

PHOs are funded to provide 'first line services' (general practice and primary nursing services), and have some flexible funding to improve access for populations with the poorest health, and funding to support health promotion. The governance group includes community representation and has responsibility to focus on the health of the enrolled population as well as build cohesion and collaboration across services and with the communities served. PHOs are not-for-profit entities, but below this umbrella structure providers can continue to operate many different models, from community-owned to small business.

A key factor in the strategy's success was timing. Against a background of falling general practice morale and income, many vibrant alternative models, particularly community-owned, Māori, and Pacific primary care services and some innovative 'mainstream' groups had developed. The strategy promised a new direction and considerable investment. It signalled a commitment to comprehensive primary health care, acknowledging general practice services as core business but requiring community participation, population health approaches, integration across services and teamwork. The need to improve health outcomes and reduce disparities had become a requirement for District Health Boards under the New Zealand Public Health & Disability Act 2000, and better primary health care was identified in the New Zealand Health Strategy as a key mechanism to achieve this (King 2000). Population-based funding and enrolled populations created opportunities to match funding to need, and enrolled populations offered the possibility of measuring impact on inequalities over time. For the first time in New Zealand, primary care would have 'a denominator', with enrolment requiring demographic characteristics of age, gender, ethnicity, locality, and deprivation level explicit for each provider and PHO. As funding was linked to this information, data quality quickly improved and was supported by national systems and audited.[2]

There were new 'structures' but 'Primary Health Organisations' were a vehicle, not an end in themselves. There was room to accommodate and build on the variety of primary care developments already in place – including the innovative 'niche' services, traditional general practice, and quality and organisational initiatives within IPAs – and to expand roles for nurse practitioners, primary care nurses, and other professionals within primary care teams. The direction was to move away from competition and managerialism to a more collaborative approach, and the expectation of a population health approach meant that creative partnerships to work on the 'big issues' across sectors could be encouraged.

An intervention framework for reducing health inequalities, based on work by Professor J. Mackenbach, was used in the National Health Committee's 1998 report (National Advisory Committee on Health and Disability 1998). It describes four levels of intervention. First, there are the underlying social and economic determinants such as income and education. At level two are the factors that are intermediate between these determinants and health (for example, work environment, smoking, nutrition, and physical activity). At level three the focus is on health and disability services – access, redistributing health resources, ensuring interventions that have a good evidence-base reach those currently missing out, developing innovative approaches, and addressing health service deficiencies. Finally, at level four, the focus is on the effect of ill health on socio-economic position (for example, job loss due to chronic illness).

This framework reflects an international drive to ensure environmental and social determinants of health – such as housing, income, and employment – receive proper attention, given the evidence of limited effectiveness of investment in medical services and vertical programmes in achieving 'Health for All' by the year 2000 (World Health Organization 2002).

By the end of the 1990s, there was considerable debate in New Zealand public health and policy circles about the optimal balance between social and economic determinants on the one hand, and health system intervention on the other, in influencing inequalities. Warnings are found in the NHC report against focusing on health services because this

> shifts the focus from underlying determinants, such as poor housing or low income, and there is only limited potential for the health sector to reduce inequalities if the fundamental determinants are ignored. (National Advisory Committee on Health and Disability 1998 : 60)

However, the Primary Health Care strategy avoids this problem of focusing on health services alone. It does so by bringing together all the elements of the four levels in Mackenbach's model (or the Ottawa Charter) in a cohesive way. The strategy is as much about intersectoral work across health organisations, government agencies, and community groups on healthy housing projects, for example, as it is about general practice and nursing services. PHOs are charged with working with communities and with other agencies to address significant population health issues. Hence, in the Capital & Coast District Health Board, the spectrum of activity that can impact on inequalities at all four levels of Mackenbach's model are in evidence. Many primary health providers already had a strong history of action in a social justice model. Others are developing the capacity to tackle structural issues at a community and political level. Advocacy for individuals across a variety of agencies is starting to be 'core' primary care business.

At this stage, the New Zealand primary care sector is still in transition from a market model to a more collaborative model. This shift involves clusters of health and social service providers working together in PHOs with iwi and communities to provide more accessible primary care services and support for preventing illness and disease, as well as for promoting good health. Although there are examples of early success, particularly in the rapid rate of PHO enrolments, there are important implementation issues that require attention if the strategy is to reduce inequalities. In the following sections, the four levels of intervention in Mackenbach's framework are used to outline positive progress in this direction, as well as potential issues.

## Underlying social and economic determinants

Several health services have included action on structural determinants as an integral part of their health service activity for many years – for example, action on income and housing issues, submissions, and political engagement. Māori providers, for instance, have worked as part of iwi (tribal authority) organisations that are involved in environmental issues, economic development, and whānau development as well as health service delivery. The Primary

Health Care strategy recognises, legitimises, and reinforces this level of action as an integral part of primary health care.

During the first year of PHO establishment, three important developments were observed. First, there has been more collective action on structural determinants at an organisational level. One example is a joint project involving the Capital & Coast District Health Board (C&CDHB) and Work and Income (W&I) with several community organisations to address marked ethnic disparities in access to discretionary benefits such as disability allowances and supplementary grants. A working group involving PHOs and other agencies has a programme with several work-streams to change inequalities in access to income support and employment. Beneath the level of the district working group, PHOs are undertaking their own initiatives to build local relationships with particular W&I staff, and are getting more involved in advocacy for individuals who experience difficulties.

Second, the flexible funding to improve access, 'Services to Improve Access' (SIA) funding, has increased the number of nurses and community health workers working outside the usual clinical settings of general practice. There are more nurses in homes, where they can see at first-hand the real barriers people are facing, and then facilitate change by making the appropriate links with government agencies and social services.

The third area is at the intersection of public health and primary health care. The funding for 'Health Promotion' is minimal at around two dollars per enrolled PHO member per year. However, PHOs have embraced the requirement and opportunity. Health Promotion planning has forged good links with the Regional Public Health Service and communities most affected by inequalities. Māori-led and Pacific-led planning is happening. The understanding that health promotion is not a contract but a paradigm is becoming more widely understood. The conventional primary care emphasis on individual lifestyle education is beginning to give way to more sophisticated analyses. There is a broader understanding that health promotion seeks to help people and communities increase control over their health. While health promotion encourages the development of personal skills, the emphasis is on working with communities rather than 'on' them, and influencing policies and decisions that will achieve health-supportive environments. It is in the area of social and economic determinants that primary care providers engage most with communities, with other sectors, with NGOs, and with local government.

## Intermediate factors

The primary care sector has always acted on the intermediate factors between social determinants and health outcomes, such as the work environment, smoking, nutrition, and physical activity. However, the inequalities focus has given more prominence to the connections between environmental factors and so-called lifestyle choices. Hence, there are examples of coalitions working to influence health options at multiple levels.

Nutrition and physical activity are a popular focus for PHOs, and funding has been dedicated to implementing the Healthy Eating – Healthy Action strategy (Ministry of Health 2003a)[3] at primary care (or community) level. The Porirua Health Cluster involves Porirua City Council, Porirua Healthlinks, Ngati Toa, Regional Public Health, Sport Wellington Region, Māori and Pacific providers, and the two Porirua PHOs. This group is working with retail outlets to ensure healthy food options are offered, promoting physical activity through local papers, and influencing recreation policy and entry charges to recreational facilities as well as monitoring progress with diabetes detection and management.

In traditional primary care, 'addressing occupational aspects of health' is usually limited to interaction with employers about an individual worker's fitness to work. There have also been some isolated but spectacular examples of organised intervention on health and safety issues, particularly by union health services. Examples include action to improve conditions and safety for refugee workers with English as a second language, and working with bus drivers to change the food and exercise options in their central depot. Such interventions are complex and often politically difficult. Getting people into employment is a fairly acceptable activity but tackling employers about employee rights, and bringing their attention to critical health and safety issues affecting vulnerable low-paid workers requires particular skill. PHO infrastructure presents health professionals with an opportunity to give more frequent consideration to workplaces as a setting for health promotion and health improvement.

## The effect of ill health on socio-economic position

Primary care providers regularly support individuals and families by facilitating income support, completing relevant forms, and advocating for more timely health interventions for people with chronic illness. There has been excellent work in the primary health care, NGO, and voluntary sectors for several years to reduce barriers to income, employment and appropriate support for people living with mental illness in the Wellington district, including outreach primary health care programmes and consumer-led initiatives.

New projects, like PATHS (Providing Access to Health Solutions) in Counties Manukau, offer intensive support in health and employment sectors for people with chronic health problems and could be effective in reducing inequalities. In all cases, the impact on inequalities depends on how the programme is implemented. As this service 'rolls out', will people with drug and alcohol dependence be in the 'too hard' basket, or will the programme offer a level of support they have not had before? Will people with high levels of education and skills benefit most, or those with co-morbidities, low income and needing significant vocational support? Primary care sensitivity to the inequalities focus will influence who is referred, who is regarded as 'eligible', and who might be offered this high-level support and flexibly funded intervention. Maintaining an inequalities focus in the implementation and evaluation of PATHS is essential to ensure this innovative service reaches those most affected by the potentially compounding effects of low income and chronic illness or disability.

## Health and disability services

Health and disability services receive constant attention from funders and the public. Despite the National Health Committee warning that this area detracts from the hard stuff, the delivery of these services is an important level of intervention. The inverse care law, which states that the availability of medical care varies inversely with the need for medical care in the population (Hart 1971), is alive and well in New Zealand. Without a determined effort to reduce inequalities within the service delivery component of primary care, there is a high risk that millions of dollars will be invested and current inequalities embedded. Those with the poorest health often have the most to gain from accessible, high quality, effective health and disability services. Furthermore, measures to improve access, such as reducing cost barriers, can be implemented relatively quickly and the effect on inequalities (for example, in service utilisation patterns) can be monitored more readily than actions at other levels of intervention.

International studies and New Zealand evidence has demonstrated that even low co-payments for primary care services are a significant barrier for many people, affecting those with poorest health the most (National Health Committee 2000). The PHC strategy signals a move to free or low cost access to primary care. In 'access-funded' PHOs and practices, the cost barrier has been reduced first (see Crampton, Chapter 10, for a description of PHO funding), with low cost access for the majority of people attending 'interim' practices being the next stage. Nationally, the effectiveness of low cost services in improving access is starting to be captured. The effectiveness of Māori providers in reducing access barriers has shown up clearly in recent reports (Ministry of Health 2004).

In the Wellington district, the inverse care law is apparent when 'utilisation' levels by ethnicity or by socio-economic status are considered, and the recipients of the services ascertained. Useful utilisation data across all providers is starting to be obtained, which means a baseline for future comparisons can be formed. It takes considerable resource and goodwill from providers to get accurate data, to include utilisation/access outside conventional clinic settings, and to agree on what analysis is relevant.

Comparative analysis based on the first attempts is superficial. It is difficult to capture the levels of complexity being dealt with, given different population groups within the same PHO and in different PHOs. Groups with high and complex needs, like refugee families, people with mental illness and other co-morbidities, people with diabetes and three or four other co-morbidities all have a higher level of complexity. The measures of 'need' in the PHO information system, which are based on age, ethnicity, and socio-economic status (using the NZDep Index of deprivation), do not enable identification of all sub-populations with higher needs.

Nevertheless, at some level and with caveats explicit, comparative analysis of available data is useful to track progress on inequalities. At a district level, for example, the population size is sufficient to overcome the limitations of a small-area measure of socio-economic status, as is the case with the NZDep Index, as well as the effect of inter-district flows. At a PHO level, feedback of this analysis keeps an 'inequalities' perspective alive. This, along with other sources of information, including input from the communities concerned, creates opportunities for more attention to equity in PHO planning. Fine-tuning is still needed in terms of resource allocation, however. Unfortunately, in terms of addressing inequalities, the funding at macro level with PHOs does not yet reflect the policy direction, as illustrated below.

Figure 11.1 summarises funding patterns for C&CDHB's five PHOs. This summary is not intended as a criticism of particular PHOs, but simply illustrates a trend observed across the country. PHOs with the highest proportion of high-needs patients have not gained as much from PHO funding as those PHOs where lower proportions of Māori, Pacific, and low-income people are enrolled. For example, Porirua Health Plus, with the highest proportion of high-needs members, has the third-largest percentage increase. The clustering of high-needs populations around particular providers and in particular PHOs is not recognised in the funding approach. The funding formula, based on historical utilisation patterns for 'first-line services' (general practice), is heavily weighted to people over 65 years and others who have traditionally accessed primary care more frequently. This funding stream has no weighting for Māori, Pacific, or low-income populations in the funding formula. Hence, the largest funding stream embeds historical inequalities.

The next phases of funding may reinforce this inequality, as major increases are for remaining age groups not currently receiving additional subsidy in 'interim PHOs', with lower percentages (although sometimes large numbers) of high needs population.

A further observation is that although the strategy is about disease prevention, health promotion, and reducing inequalities through services addressing unmet needs, by far the most funding is dedicated to 'first-line services' – that is, general practice consultation. This is illustrated in Figure 11.2. In the funding streams for health promotion and 'Services to Improve Access' there is a small weighting (0.2) for Māori, Pacific, and low-income populations. This adjustment does little to acknowledge the work required to make a difference to the unequal access and health status of these sub-populations.

## Decisions within PHOs

Within PHOs there is an equally important level of decision-making. Decisions have to be made about who has priority when appointments are in demand,

|  | Based on April '04 Registers | | From 1 July '03 to 30 June '04 | | From 1 July '04 |
| --- | --- | --- | --- | --- | --- |
| PHO | Enrolled Population | % High Needs | PHO Funding | % Inc. | CPI Adjustments & 65+ Increase |
| Capital PHO | 129,297 | 12 | 7,512,902 | 73 | 1,092,768 |
| Kapiti PHO | 33,002 | 10 | 2,550,819 | 48 | 772,217 |
| Tumai mo te Iwi | 45,335 | 36 | 4,297,861 | 184 | 307,656 |
| Porirua Health Plus | 12,919 | 92 | 1,950,791 | 49 | 32,989 |
| SECPHO | 9,601 | 57 | 1,144,578 | 17 | 8,282 |

*Figure 11.1: PHO funding by PHO in Capital & Coast DHB (including comparison with previous funding under the General Medical Subsidy (GMS[4]))*

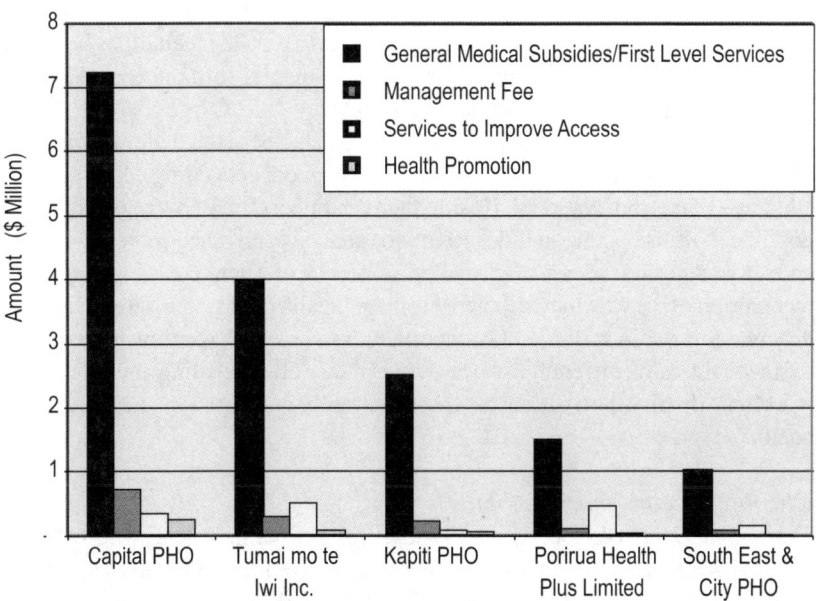

*Figure 11.2: Funding for 12 months – by health services and PHOs, 1 July 2003 to 1 July 2004*

information will be written in. These might be called 'micro-equity' decisions, but they involve the allocation of resources and are complex for all PHOs.

For Porirua Plus PHO, where the PHO population is 95 per cent Māori, Pacific, and low income, virtually any decision will impact on high-needs populations. What does reducing inequalities mean in this context? Should PHOs invest in innovative whānau models? Should they provide interpreters for refugees? The reality is that, for this PHO, the intervention required is an increase in funding and resources across the board so that they can overcome historical under-investment and continue to improve patient access and apply evidence, innovation, and community knowledge to reduce inequalities.

The large Capital PHO has a different problem, as it has or will have significant additional funding. This PHO has the greatest number of Māori, Pacific, and low-income members but they are scattered among many providers over a large area. The problem here is one of effectively redistributing resources. This raises such questions as who to engage with, how to balance the demands of a largely middle-class population who expect benefits from the new structures with the needs of Māori, Pacific, and low-income families within the same practices, and what mechanisms are needed to engender meaningful community participation in a big PHO with a diverse population.

How decisions are made and who makes them (who is 'at the table') affects inequalities. Responsibility to manage this tension and push the boundaries towards equitable resource allocation and action to reduce inequalities lies with District Health Boards as well as PHOs. Fundamental shifts need to happen, but every marginal shift progresses the agenda.

With enrolled populations, it is possible to achieve much better monitoring of how decisions impact differentially. With good geocoding, age, gender, ethnicity data, and National Health Index numbers in PHO registers, it is possible to utilise an inequalities frame for analysis and make more intelligent collective decisions about what makes a difference. There can also be greater recognition of the way in which barriers in our health care systems disadvantage different groups. In addition, it is important to pay careful attention to the effect on inequalities of different service delivery models, including the effects on workforce distribution, patient access, community participation and population health outcomes.

## Chronic disease management

There is an increasing need for chronic disease management. The original 'disease state management' models to improve care for chronic disease, based on guidelines and best practice, were implemented in a standardised way, in the belief that the benefits would be enjoyed by all. One of the most striking findings in the evaluation of 10 integrated care pilot projects, reported in 2001, was the variable impact of these well-funded projects on Māori with chronic disease. The projects which operated in a bicultural framework and had well-established relationships with local iwi, good Māori representation at all levels, and Māori well represented in the decision-making process achieved engagement in their projects. In other projects, despite reports of consulting with Māori, Māori were not involved in decision-making and a true partnership relationship did not develop (Health Services Research Centre, Te Ropu Rangahau Hauora a Eru Pomare 2001).

There is evidence of learning from the failure of generic approaches to reduce inequalities, and a growing realisation that international 'best practice' must be adapted to the New Zealand setting – in other words, we should be a little less 'colonised' in our application of evidence. Aukati kai paipa, the Māori smoking cessation programme, has taught the value of Māori-specific approaches. This programme demonstrated a 29 per cent quit rate for Māori women compared to a latent quit rate of 12.5 per cent. Point prevalence quit rate at 12 months was 23 per cent for all participants (26 per cent at 6 months) (Ministry of Health 2003b). The Sudden Infant Death Syndrome (SIDS) programmes initially took a 'generic' approach, but failed to reduce Māori rates of sudden infant death. A Māori-led approach has had a measurable effect. The value of tailored programmes using evidence but designed in partnership with the communities they affect, and led by appropriate providers, is now being recognised.

In C&CDHB there are innovative programmes, such as the retinal screening programme for people with diabetes. This service has moved out from the hospital, utilises optometrists, and works with a range of providers and across PHOs to achieve better coverage. The initiative has been successful in reducing inequalities in access to retinal screening. There are successful Māori-led asthma programmes, and a relatively low level of asthma admissions for children compared to other health board districts. There is not the same success yet with Pacific children's asthma, so differential investment is required here. However, a Pacific service, working from the hospital base, has now incorporated a Pacific primary care nurse linking back into PHOs. The service aims to reduce inequalities through active follow-up back into community and primary care settings.

There is a heart failure project, focused on Porirua, to ensure 'gold standard' care is available to those with highest morbidity. While this example is not primary care specific, by linking primary care with chronic disease management the project can influence integration and optimisation of services for people with the highest burden of ill health.

### Disability, He Korowai Oranga, PHO population size
The barriers for people with disability are also being discussed in PHOs. Some PHOs have spent considerable time looking at their own behaviours and prejudices, have undertaken disability awareness training, and are approaching accessibility in a more rigorous way to reduce this dimension of inequality. C&CDHB required NZ Disability Strategy to be reflected in business cases for PHO development, to at least signal the importance of this strategy being actively addressed in decision-making.

Improving Māori health and supporting Māori development presents a major challenge. The strengths-based paradigm of whānau ora presented in He Korowai Oranga, the Māori Health Strategy (King and Turia 2002), is an empowerment model that links with the Primary Health Care Strategy. He Korowai Oranga requires a significant shift in thinking for the health and social service sector. Having the right people 'around the table' in PHO governance and in DHB interactions creates the possibility of partnership and investment in Māori-led initiatives.

To end this section on decision-making, a comment on the size of PHO populations is relevant. As the implementation of PHOs began, a minimum size of 70,000 people was suggested by some in the Ministry of Health. The Minister decided to allow the balance between management efficiency and community-connectedness to be explored over the early implementation phase. Views have been expressed that small PHOs need to merge to gain 'economies of scale'. The interesting observation in C&CDHB is that smaller PHOs manage all the functions required of them, in the main charge less, and deliver a wide range of innovative services to populations with high and complex health needs. Providers in the smaller PHOs have a track record in working with communities, and reducing both inequalities and barriers. If the issue of costs of PHO management arises as contractual expectations grow, it can be addressed through the management fee. Nationally, there has been historical under-investment in many providers within small PHOs, while larger PHOs tend to have Independent Practitioner Association (IPA) management services that build on infrastructure, funded through budget-holding contracts over many years. The ability to perform at a corporate level may be required of PHOs, but a broader measure of their performance is also needed. In other words, accessible and affordable services, a range of services, community participation, and the ability to make a difference to inequalities are some of the dimensions to be considered along with management outputs when judging the success of PHOs, big or small.

## Conclusion

New Zealand is experiencing a climate of change with an unprecedented policy focus on reducing disparities, a formalised approach to influencing social and economic determinants of health, and a major shift in health service focus resulting in greater investment in primary health care. Reducing inequalities means differential investment. It means taking risks, supporting innovation, and tracking the effectiveness – not generally, but specifically. It means overcoming denial that the barriers, prejudice, injustice, and inequity exist and moving to change this.

The Primary Health Care Strategy is providing the mechanisms, new resources, community energy, and a revitalised sector. This chapter has emphasised that the success of this strategy in reducing inequalities will not be achieved through structures and contracts, but through a 'movement' for change. Fundamental to this is a shift in power, which includes giving more power to communities, more power-sharing within teams, shared decision-making, moving away from ownership to leadership, and stepping back to let others own and lead.

# 12. Reducing health inequalities by improving housing

Philippa Howden-Chapman and Sarah Bierre

Like employment, housing is of critical importance for a range of social and economic reasons. Decent housing is about more than having a roof over your head. The cost, quality and location of housing have a material impact on a family's well-being today and the children's prospects tomorrow (Ministry of Social Development 2005: 61).

'Housing is work, home and politics' (Dickens *et al*. 1985: 11).

It is salutary to remember that children born into low-income households will have more illness and shorter lives, on average, than those born into high-income households (Marsh *et al*. 2000; Næss *et al*. 2004). But why is this so? Do lower incomes buy less healthy housing, and do these less healthy housing conditions partially explain the difference in life chances? And, if differences in housing quality are part of the answer, is it possible to identify research-based housing interventions that can reduce these health inequalities? This chapter attempts to answer these questions and highlight what is already known about reducing health inequalities by improving housing.

Public health policy frameworks in New Zealand and elsewhere are increasingly based on the premise that it is the *unequal* distribution of social, economic, and environmental determinants of health that leads to inequalities in health, and that attempts to address health inequalities without tackling these underlying unequal distributions of resources and social conditions are likely to fail (Ministry of Health 2002). This acceptance of the premise that interconnected underlying structures such as housing, employment patterns, and income determine the pattern of health has encouraged researchers and governments to investigate ways to modify these structures, and implement changes to them, to the advantage of the less well-off (Graham 2001).

Reducing inequalities in the determinants of health has become the new public health paradigm, but there is much less consensus about whether to, or how to, make society more egalitarian. Policy debates have highlighted two main options – universal entitlements or targeted policies. Universal social policies, such as the provision of public schooling and superannuation, while efficient, are seen by many within the dominant economic discipline as less effective than targeted policies (Kuila 1993). But targeting of state housing, for example, inevitably leads to some people who are in need missing out and, frequently, those who do not miss out being stigmatised as receiving state handouts – social assistance which is denied to the majority (Murphy 1999). However, for Māori and the Crown, the provisions of the Treaty of Waitangi cut across these policy debates and carry clear expectations that issues of particular concern for Māori will be prioritised for equity reasons. Arguably, for Māori, who have had unequal access to quality housing and housing subsidies in the past, safe affordable housing is one such issue (Tennant 2004; Bierre *et al*. 2007).

Rose has highlighted the possibly unintended consequence of targeting by criticising the tendency to view marginal groups as 'problem groups, different and separate from the rest of society'. He likens some problems to icebergs whose visible tips can neither be understood nor properly controlled if they are thought to be the *whole* problem (Rose 1992: 96). Primarily relying on targeted policies can also be seen as a reductionist approach – attempting to modify the determinants of health, but addressing a minor though important part of the interlinked whole.

> Recognition of the inequities in health status associated with, for example, poverty, inadequate housing, lack of employment opportunities, racism and powerlessness has led to calls for a renewed focus on an ecological approach that recognises that individuals are embedded within social, political and economic systems that shape behaviours and access to resources necessary to maintain health. (Israel *et al*. 1998: 174)

In this chapter, housing is considered from an economic, social, and environmental perspective as a setting where potentially major redistributive policies can be designed, which may yield demonstrable improvements in health. In this context, He Kainga Oranga/Housing and Health Research Programme is highlighted as a place where housing interventions, which could have an impact on health, are tested and actively disseminated to the public and policy-makers.

## Inequalities in housing

Decent, affordable housing is not equally available to all. From an economic perspective, inadequate housing can be seen as one of the multiple consequences of low income (Le Grand *et al*. 1984). Housing represents the largest single living-cost item for most people and their largest asset, which they can use to 'smooth' their available income if required (that is, by increasing their mortgage to provide disposable income if necessary). House prices in New Zealand have increased significantly over the last decade (faster than inflation) and the rate of home ownership has fallen, from 74 per cent in 1989 to 66.9 per cent in 2006 (Thomson 1991; Statistics New Zealand 2007). Overall, there has been a substantial increase since the late 1980s in the proportion of households spending more than 30 per cent of their income on housing (Ministry of Social Development 2005), yet indications from surveys are that most people in rental properties would still like to own their own home, both for security and as a way of improving the quality of their housing (Robinson 2005).

With the rapid rise in the proportion of households renting, the availability of decent rental housing has become problematic. Information problems faced by new arrivals to urban areas in particular are often exacerbated by ethnic or other forms of discrimination, which prevent them from obtaining housing outside narrowly defined areas. As a result, people in a more deprived neighbourhood can pay a higher price per unit than other people pay for good quality housing in less economically deprived neighbourhoods (Le Grand *et al.* 1984). Indeed, stock-takes of housing quality have consistently highlighted the under-investment in housing in areas where there are more Māori households (National Housing Commission 1988).

More Māori and low-income people rent both in the private rental market and in social housing, and there is repeated evidence of racial discrimination in the former (MacDonald 1986; National Housing Commission 1988; Waldegrave *et al.* 2000). Studies have indicated a 'gate-keeper' (Spoonley 1975) mentality in the housing market, where barriers are put up to restrict the property available for Māori and Pacific peoples in comparison to Pākehā. Landlords and real estate agents are more likely to tell Māori and Pacific peoples that houses are no longer available, to quote higher rental prices, to invent conditions making them ineligible, and divert attempts made to express interest in property. Māori are often directed or forced to take up lower quality or state housing, even where income levels were adequate for a higher quality house (Māori Women's Housing Research Project 1991). Indeed, a recent report of self-reported racial discrimination on Māori health and inequalities found that the most marked inequality was in buying and renting housing, where Māori were 13 times more likely to report being treated unfairly because of their ethnicity than were Europeans (Harris *et al.* 2006).

Traditional patterns of land ownership, individually owned in a capitalist society and communally owned in a tribal society, have advantaged Pākehā in New Zealand society (Belgrave 2004; McClure 2004). Indeed, W.H. Oliver has argued that the New Zealand Company's system of purchasing Māori land and reselling the land to settlers was the first instrument of social policy in New Zealand (Oliver 1988). Nineteenth-century Pākehā 'enablement' was thus predicated on the dispossession of communally owned land from Māori. Individual title makes it easier to meet or overcome restrictions imposed by various land-use planning laws and to raise a mortgage and achieve home ownership, and this has remained a significant factor in Pākehā achieving higher levels of home ownership than Māori. Moreover, there is a remarkable absence of a wealth, capital gains tax or estate duties in New Zealand, exceptional in the OECD states. These factors have led to a greater proportion of older

Pākehā people compared to older Māori people being home-owners. Often by retirement Pākehā own their home without a mortgage, which combined with their ability to realise untaxed capital gains from the houses they or their parents have owned, leads to a greater concentration of wealth.

Yet, there are a group of disadvantaged households who live in temporary accommodation which they neither own nor rent. A recent qualitative study of people living in temporary accommodation has found that, though for some it is their preferred state, for others such accommodation is a result of ill health and lack of availability of affordable housing (Dew & Carroll 2007 ). While New Zealand has unusually low levels of homelessness (National Housing Commission 1988), there is a corollary problem of crowding (Howden-Chapman & Wilson 2000). Although, overall, this particular problem is diminishing, in 2002 approximately 10 per cent of the New Zealand population lived in households requiring one or more additional bedrooms (Ministry of Social Development 2005) and some regions have experienced increased crowding over time (Widmer 2006).

## Government interventions to supply housing

Over the lifetime of the New Zealand welfare state, housing policy has shifted from more interventionist economic thinking focusing on supply-side policies to a neoclassical demand-side emphasis (Thorns 2000). The state has experimented with supplying low-cost state-owned, quality affordable housing, as well as increasing demand through the allocation of financial assistance to those on low incomes to enable them to increase their purchasing power in either the rental or home-ownership market (Murphy & Kearns 1994). The New Zealand Treasury argued strongly from the mid-1980s that an indirect system of income supplementation was preferable to a direct system of income-related housing benefits (New Zealand Treasury 1984, 1987, 1990).

A key policy of the early welfare state was to offer interest-free grants and low-interest mortgages to young adults seeking to buy their own homes, but this policy, which was initially universally available to all families, became increasingly targeted. From the early 1990s, the focus of housing assistance has been on direct financial support for eligible low-income persons, in rental or mortgaged property. An accommodation benefit was put in place, later replaced by a less restricted supplement that was both means and asset-tested. Income-related rents replaced market-rated rents for tenants of state-owned houses in 2001, following the election of a Labour-led coalition.

Reflecting the changes in the prevailing philosophy of the leading political party of the time, the target for social housing, constructed by the state, has also changed from 'the worker and his family' to a focus on those who are deemed to be in highest need of safe, 'affordable' housing, and for whom the market system of allocating houses has serious shortcomings. By the early 1960s the stock of state houses was around 60,000 and they formed about 10 per cent of the national housing stock (Thomson et al. 2001). In 2006, while the number of state and local authority rented houses is approximately the same, this stock now forms less than 5 per cent of the overall housing stock and is amongst the smallest proportion in the OECD (Ministry of Social Policy 2005). Indeed the proportion of social housing or not-for profit housing in New Zealand is considerably less than the 20 per cent social housing in the UK and levels in Switzerland, Germany, Austria, and Sweden, where a majority of the renting population rent from social, or not-for profit, landlords (Ambrose & Nicholson 2004).

Governments have increasingly focused housing assistance towards those most in need, as distinct from a situation 'where benefits are directed at people with specific needs' (Thorns 1988). One of the consequences in the 1960s and 1970s was the creation of low-income suburbs, a result of policy that targeted low-income families for state housing assistance, together with geographically grouping these houses in set-aside areas, such as Otara, Mangere, and Porirua. The Housing Act 1955 was 'concerned with building houses, not with the concept of creating total communities, which would include the provision of desirable and necessary amenities and services' (Trlin 1977: 129).

With the growth of suburbia and the narrowing of the grounds of eligibility for state housing came a new stigma (Shrader 2005). Using income as an indicator of need meant that single-parent families were accepted as tenants more often than usual, as were Māori and Pacific Island peoples (Ferguson 1994). Because overall New Zealand has such a low proportion of social housing, the social allocation model means that tenants selected usually have multiple social, economic, and health disadvantages (Baker et al. forthcoming). With increasingly selective targeting, the incipient trend to residential segregation is currently being reinforced by property developers placing covenants on land titles in order to keep state-housing tenants out of newly established neighbourhoods (Gregory 2006).

## Housing and health problems

Owners of older homes are more likely to be people on low incomes, as new homes and apartments are more likely to be owner-occupied, and first-home buyers on low incomes tend to buy older homes (Thomson et al. 1991). As rates of home-ownership have fallen, there has, not surprisingly, been a fall in the number of low-income households who have been able to afford to buy their own home.

Older homes and rental dwellings are likely to be harder to heat due to inefficient or inadequate heating systems, poor construction, and lack of insulation. People on low incomes are also more likely to be in more crowded accommodation and sometimes, as in the case of older people, in properties that are too large for their needs and thus difficult and expensive to heat. The widespread use of unflued gas heaters in New Zealand, along with second-hand smoke, adds to indoor air pollution which causes respiratory and other problems (Garrett et al. 1998; Thomson et al. 2005; Howden-Chapman et al. 2007).

When households have to spend more than 10 per cent of their total household income on all household fuels to achieve a satisfactory indoor environment, they are considered to be suffering from fuel poverty (Healy 2004). Lloyd ( 2006) has calculated that between 10 per cent and 14 per cent of households are in fuel poverty in New Zealand. People on low incomes may try and manage fuel bills by cutting back on fuel, but this can lead to cold and damp conditions that encourage mould, which can in turn cause asthma and exacerbate respiratory problems. The combination of high rainfall and fuel poverty may be a reason why about a third of New Zealand householders report significant mould problems (Howden-Chapman *et al*. 2005).

New Zealand is unusual because, although it is a temperate country, there is a high level of excess winter mortality (Davie 2004). This, as in Ireland and Portugal, is likely to be related to housing standards and heating (Healy 2004). The problem is a significant one in New Zealand, where it is estimated that there about 1600 excess deaths each winter (Davie 2004).

There is a high level of personal indebtedness in New Zealand, and among low-income people the debt is disproportionately owed to the state. If low-income households try and maintain adequate levels of warmth, their general level of indebtedness can rise; to avoid this, they cut back on other essential items such as food and clothing. Discussing the rationale for whether benefit levels should be calculated before or after the inclusion of housing costs, Ambrose and Nicholson provide a graphic picture of the trade-offs families on low incomes often make:

> But who pays the rent and council tax is not the issue. It has to be paid and there is no margin for error, official mistakes or a crisis in statutory minimum incomes. Deprivation is a life of threats. Eviction for rent arrears; a fine or prison for council tax, TV licence arrears and truancy; disconnection for gas, electricity and BT [telephone] arrears; and bailiffs for all of them, make deprived families, struggling to pay for food, for school clothing, vulnerable to the extortionate interest rate of door-to-door lenders and catalogue companies. There is no punishment, but ill health and anxiety, for cutting down on food, fuel and clothes. (2004: 12)

Faced with issues of declining home ownership, declining rates of social housing, poorly insulated and unsafely heated homes, damp and mouldy homes, pockets of crowding, and serious housing need, the research challenge is to identify housing interventions that will address these issues, all of which are linked to poor health outcomes, and can reduce inequalities in health (Howden-Chapman *et al*. 2004).

While systematic reviews have shown that few controlled studies have demonstrated the causal link between housing and health, a number of promising studies have been highlighted (Thomson *et al*. 2001): the positive effects of rehousing based on medical need, installing energy efficiency measures, housing improvement in the context of area or community regeneration, and refurbishment and renovation. The next section describes a research programme designed to fill the gap these authors identify by undertaking 'large scale studies that investigate the wider social context of housing improvements and their comparative effectiveness and cost effectiveness' (Thomson *et al.* 2001: 189).

Timely research that addresses the local context and collaboratively links the academic and policy-making community is likely to have more influence in informing policy (Davis & Howden-Chapman 1996). In addition, evaluations are more influential if they are commissioned by the relevant ministries, are based on the local collection of data, and instruments and incentives to implement policy are available. He Kainga Oranga/Housing and Health Research Programme was deliberately set up to take account of these factors.

## He Kainga Oranga/Housing and Health Research Programme

In 2001, He Kainga Oranga/Housing and Health Research Programme gained funding from the Health Research Council of New Zealand and a number of other public and private funders for the express purpose of generating knowledge to reduce inequalities in health by addressing the quality and availability of housing in New Zealand (Howden-Chapman *et al.* 2004).[1] The aim of the programme is to establish causal links between housing and health, which can lead to a firm evidence base for this link and encourage more cross-sectoral investment in this area. Every effort has been made to work in partnership with local community organisations, so that they can help set the agenda and reap the benefits, principally from the interventions, but also potentially from opportunities for employment and community development (Matheson *et al.* 2005).

Two flagship projects were set up: the Housing, Insulation and Health Study (Howden-Chapman *et al.* 2005) and the Housing, Crowding and Health Study (Baker *et al.* 2004). Subsequently, the research programme has been funded to undertake the Housing, Heating and Health Study and the Housing and (Dis)ability Study, an exploratory study of institutional factors that can influence housing modifications. Each study addresses a key health policy issue and has been designed to provide clear evidence of effective policies.

## The Housing, Insulation and Health Study

The indoor environment in New Zealand housing is several degrees colder than recommended by the World Health Organization (1987). There are a variety of reasons for this: our climate is temperate, but has a high rainfall which leads to high relative humidity, which makes the air more difficult to warm; about a third of houses were built before insulation was required by the Building Code; and culturally New Zealanders have a preference for heating only one room of their house (Isaacs 2005).

To answer the policy question about whether installing retrofit insulation increases the indoor temperature and improves the health of the household, the Housing, Insulation and Health Study was carried out. It was an ambitious community-based trial of almost 1400 households, in which there was at least one person suffering from respiratory symptoms and where the house was uninsulated.

The study was carried out in partnership with eight locally based organisations in different parts of New Zealand. The intervention involved the retrofitting of houses with the standard insulation package developed by the government Energy Efficiency and Conservation Authority. Local people were employed as interviewers and to work in teams to retrofit the houses (Howden-Chapman et al. 2005). Almost half the people in the study identified as Māori and a quarter as Pacific people. Results showed that insulating older houses led to a small but significant rise in the indoor temperature and a drop in relative humidity (Howden-Chapman et al. 2005; Howden-Chapman et al. 2007). These changes in the indoor environment were sufficient to lead to both subjectively and objectively measured improvements in people's well-being and health: they had fewer days off school and work, fewer days in hospital, and they used 23 per cent less energy to heat their houses.

A cost-benefit study showed that benefits were greater than the costs by a substantial margin (about 1.6 to 1) (Chapman et al. submitted). Moreover, some evidence suggests it is not a misunderstanding of the benefits of insulation that stands in households' way of installing it; given that households express realistic 'willingness to pay' for insulation, other factors such as the landlord/tenant incentive problems and household cash constraints may be key barriers (O'Dea et al. 2006). Since the preliminary publication of these study results, considerable efforts have been made by the research team to disseminate them, and this has led to significantly increased government expenditure on home insulation, which has been dispersed to local community organisations (Howden-Chapman unpublished).

As a follow-up to the Insulation Study, 400 households in which there is a child between six and twelve years of age who has doctor-diagnosed asthma, and where the form of household heating is either an unflued gas heater or a plug-in electric heater, have been enrolled in the Housing, Heating and Health Study (Howden-Chapman et al. 2005). As the Insulation Study found that the retrofitted insulation raised the temperature of the house only about a degree or less, the intervention in this study involves both insulating the houses *and* installing more powerful heaters that do not pollute the indoor environment, use sustainable forms of heating, and have the capacity to heat more of the house. Objective and subjective measures of health, health services, energy consumption, and the indoor environment were again measured in the winter of 2005 and, following the installation of insulation and new heaters in a randomly allocated half of the houses, follow-up measures were taken in the winter of 2006. The results showed a significant increase in temperature and reduction in asthma symptoms (Howden-Chapman et al. submitted)

# The Housing, Crowding and Health Study

Household crowding has long been recognised as a major risk factor for infectious diseases (Baker *et al*. 2000; McNicholas *et al*. 2000; Baker *et al*. forthcoming). However, for low-income families, it has been difficult to tell whether it is low household income or crowding that is the main cause of an infection spreading. This is an important policy question, because if household crowding can be reduced through welfare benefits or the taxation regime, the need for government intervention in the housing market would be less urgent.

As discussed previously, New Zealand governments have recognised the importance of supporting social housing, even though the level of that support is considerably lower here than in European countries. The current justification is to supply safe, affordable housing for those on low incomes and with high social needs. In consequence of the highly targeted social allocation model, which recognises the extent of the economic deprivation of the Māori and Pacific Island communities (Howden-Chapman & Tobias 2000; Blakely *et al*. 2002) and the discriminatory private rental market, two-thirds of Housing New Zealand Corporation (HNZC) tenants are either Māori or Pacific Islanders.

The Housing, Crowding and Health Study, which began in 2003, is an ongoing cohort study of all applicant and tenant households applying to or renting from HNZC. HNZC administrative data on individual households are linked to individuals' hospitalisation records. The aim of the study is to see whether tenants live in less crowded circumstances than applicants, and whether this reduction in overcrowding – if it occurs – reduces episodes of hospitalisation (Baker *et al*. 2004; Baker & Zhang 2005). Interim reports have shown that housing applicants have larger households and higher levels of crowding than tenants, but both groups have higher crowding levels than the average New Zealand household (Baker & Zhang 2005). However, the majority (60 per cent) of applicants who become tenants markedly reduce their level of household crowding in the process (Turner *et al*. 2004). Furthermore, tenants have significantly fewer episodes of hospitalisation than applicants (Baker & Zhang 2005). These results would suggest that providing state housing serves the government's stated purpose of improving low-income people's living circumstances, which leads to an improvement in their health that in turn reduces the need for hospitalisation.

# The Tokelau Extended-Family Study

In addition to the community trials and the cohort study of state tenants, the Tokelau Extended-Family Study grew out of a partnership with the Wellington Tokelau Association. A series of focus groups was held to understand the Tokelau community's view of the impact of housing on health, in particular their view of crowding (Howden-Chapman *et al*. 2000). Although cultural patterns are an essential part of Tokelau hospitality, the decision to 'double up' households is often the result of 'rational' economic decision-making in relation to household expenditures such as rent and food. The implication for public health practitioners is that while overcrowding in existing state housing may be a health hazard for residents, the most effective solutions for the community are higher household income and more flexible housing designs that accommodate multi-family households.

These focus groups were followed by a random survey of Tokelau families about household expenditure (Pene *et al.* 2002). Since then, a community action project has been designed, which involves working with community architects to build one new purpose-designed extended-family house and refurbish an old one in Eastern Porirua, which is the site of a Housing New Zealand Corporation community renewal programme. These new, more spacious houses will be evaluated after the extended families move in to assess the impact on the health and well-being of family members. Building commenced in 2007 and is being accompanied by a pre- and post-occupancy evaluation.

## The Healthy Housing Index

The Healthy Housing Index has been conceived as a 'warrant of fitness' measure of housing quality that could be widely used to draw attention to the aspects of New Zealand homes that may contribute to ill health or accidents. It is based on the British House Condition Survey and combines evidence from housing and health research and building science (Bierre *et al.* 2004). It is being piloted in the Hutt Valley with co-funding from the local city council and District Health Board as well as the Accident Compensation Corporation (ACC), and showed that the number of hazards in the house significantly predicted the number of injury claims (Keall *et al.* forthcoming). The Index is now being rolled out in Taranaki to appraise injury hazards in a thousand houses as a prelude to a major intervention study to reduce home injuries. It is planned to further develop the index as a Whānau Ora tool for use by Māori, at a whānau or iwi level, to appraise the quality of their housing in terms of any health problems experienced by residents, and recommend improvements. The Index has the potential to be used as either a regulatory tool to enforce overall housing standards, as a tool for community improvement, as a way of signalling to the market the housing features that enhance health, or as an indicator to landlords of desirable repairs.

## Conclusion

Housing is a key, if recently neglected, determinant of health and health inequalities. Yet, it is a readily available setting for a number of demonstrably effective public health interventions. Responding to the international interest in more robust evidence to inform policy, He Kainga Oranga/Housing and Health Research Programme has shown that, by carrying out community trials, cohort studies, and community action programmes, clearer causal links between housing and health can be established, and practical interventions can be trialled and more widely implemented. These projects have supported the case for more cross-sectoral investment in healthy housing, and emphasised the broader social benefits ('external' to the housing market) of improving the quality of housing.

Subsidising the retrofitted insulation of older houses is a good social and economic investment that pays dividends at an individual, household, and community level. The ready availability of social housing can reduce levels of crowding and the rates of hospitalisation among low-income families. These results suggest that providing state housing serves the purpose of improving low-income people's living circumstances. This leads to an improvement in the health of household members and reduces the demand for hospitalisation. Thus better living circumstances and healthier housing reduces the burden of low income and poor health that the household previously had to carry. More generally, communities have clear ideas about the features of their housing and built environment that increase their health and well-being. He Kainga Oranga/Housing and Health Research Programme has highlighted the fact that community organisations are often well-informed and articulate, and, given the opportunity, can ably work in partnership with researchers and policy people to develop and implement these ideas.

# 13. Tools for health equity

## Louise Signal

Tools or aids to practice such as guidelines, frameworks, and checklists are used in many spheres to guide policy, programme or service development, implementation, and evaluation. Two health equity tools, the *Intervention Framework to Improve Health and Reduce Inequalities* (Intervention Framework) (Ministry of Health 2002) and the *Health Equity Assessment Tool* (HEAT tool) (Ministry of Health *et al.* 2004) have been recently used across the New Zealand health sector, with some success, to assist in tackling inequalities in health. They were developed as part of an initiative by the Ministry of Health (MoH) to strengthen the capacity of the health sector to address health inequalities.

This chapter explains the tools, discusses training in their use, and reviews their application and value in the New Zealand health sector. It takes a social approach to the causes of inequalities in health, reflecting the shift in international literature in recent years away from biological explanations to an examination of social factors (Krieger 2001). This position is consistent with that of Graham (Graham 2001), who argues that inequalities arise from, and are maintained by, the unequal distribution of the determinants of health – in other words, the unequal distribution of factors such as income, employment, education, housing, health care, and social support. It is the privileging of some people and groups over others, by factors such as race, class, gender, geography or 'ableism',[1] that generates social inequalities.

The concepts of 'social inequalities in health' and 'social inequities in health' are used interchangeably in this chapter and are defined as:

> health disparities, within and between countries, that are judged to be unfair, unjust, avoidable, and unnecessary (meaning: are neither inevitable nor unremediable) that systematically burden populations rendered vulnerable by underlying social structures and political, economic, and legal institutions (Krieger 2001).

Inequalities in health and in the determinants of health are pronounced in New Zealand. They include inequalities between ethnic groups, people of different socio-economic status, geographic inequalities, inequalities of gender, and inequalities experienced by people with disabilities (Minister for Disability Issues 2001; Ministry of Health 2002).

Of particular concern are the large and persistent inequalities experienced by Māori, which increased throughout the 1980s and 1990s. Pacific people also experienced a widening inequalities gap over this period (Ajwani *et al*. 2003). While absolute socio-economic inequalities in mortality were stable during this time, there was an increase in relative socio-economic inequalities[2] (Blakely *et al*. 2005). Inequalities in health are not a biological given. They are the unfair and unjust result of social and economic policy and practice. Therefore, just as inequalities have developed so they can be reduced (Woodward and Kawachi 2000).

The recent Labour-led governments have made a commitment to reduce inequalities in health, education, employment, and housing. This commitment is one of the six key government goals to guide public sector policy and performance. The over-arching New Zealand Health Strategy, which sets the platform for the government's action on health, acknowledges the need to address health inequalities as 'a major priority requiring ongoing commitment across the sector' (Ministry of Health 2000).

This chapter explores how health equity tools can assist the health sector to meet this commitment to reduce inequalities in health. These tools may also be useful in other sectors with a significant impact on health, well-being, and equity. The discussion here is based on the author's experience in developing the HEAT tool (Ministry of Health *et al*. 2004), in applying both tools, in training health sector workers in the use of the tools (Carroll *et al*. 2004), and in reviewing the application of the tools in the New Zealand health sector (Signal & Martin 2005).

# The tools

## *The intervention framework*

The Intervention Framework (Ministry of Health 2002) provides a guide for the development and implementation of comprehensive strategies to improve health and tackle inequalities in health (see Figure 13.1). It identifies many contributing social factors that need to be addressed. It indicates that solutions to inequalities in health lie across many sectors, and require comprehensive packages of policies and interventions (Mackenbach *et al*. 2002). In addition, the Intervention Framework provides a way of conceptualising the range of factors. The framework identifies that, to make a significant difference to the health of populations, comprehensive strategies must be developed that target all four of the following areas.

*Structural strategies* tackle the root causes of health inequalities, namely the social, economic, cultural, and historical factors that fundamentally determine health. Specific examples of action include systematic implementation of the provisions of the Treaty of Waitangi in policy, programme, and service delivery; monitoring health inequalities and social determinants; and policies that ensure equitable education, labour market, housing, and other social outcomes.

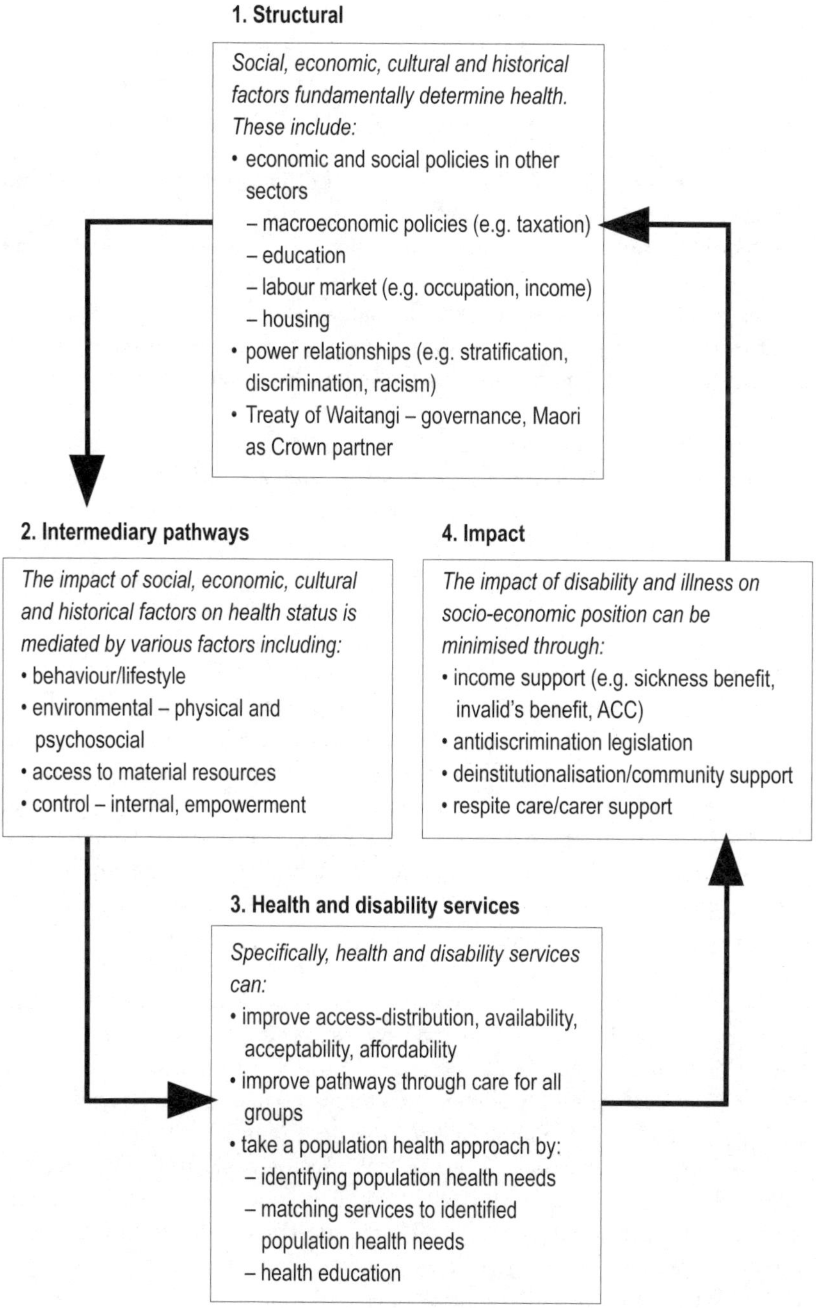

**1. Structural**

*Social, economic, cultural and historical factors fundamentally determine health. These include:*
- economic and social policies in other sectors
  - macroeconomic policies (e.g. taxation)
  - education
  - labour market (e.g. occupation, income)
  - housing
- power relationships (e.g. stratification, discrimination, racism)
- Treaty of Waitangi – governance, Maori as Crown partner

**2. Intermediary pathways**

*The impact of social, economic, cultural and historical factors on health status is mediated by various factors including:*
- behaviour/lifestyle
- environmental – physical and psychosocial
- access to material resources
- control – internal, empowerment

**4. Impact**

*The impact of disability and illness on socio-economic position can be minimised through:*
- income support (e.g. sickness benefit, invalid's benefit, ACC)
- antidiscrimination legislation
- deinstitutionalisation/community support
- respite care/carer support

**3. Health and disability services**

*Specifically, health and disability services can:*
- improve access-distribution, availability, acceptability, affordability
- improve pathways through care for all groups
- take a population health approach by:
  - identifying population health needs
  - matching services to identified population health needs
  - health education

Interventions at each level may apply: nationally, regionally and locally; taking population and individual approaches

*Figure 13.1: Intervention framework to improve health and reduce inequalities*

*Intermediary pathway* strategies target material, psychosocial, and behavioural factors that mediate the impact of structural factors on health. Specific examples of action include community development programmes, local authority policies, and settings-based programmes such as healthy cities and health-promoting schools.

*Health and disability services* undertake specific actions within health and disability services. Examples include improved access to appropriate, higher-quality health care and disability services; ethnic-specific service delivery; and collaborative partnerships within the health sector and intersectorally.

*Impact* focuses on minimising the impact of disability and illness on socio-economic position. Specific examples of action include income support, disability allowance, and antidiscrimination legislation and education.

The Intervention Framework combines a model of the social and economic determinants of health developed by Howden-Chapman and Tobias (Howden-Chapman & Tobias 2000) with an intervention framework developed by Johan Mackenbach of Erasmus University (pers. comm. cited in National Health Committee 1998). It is presented in the MoH publication *Reducing Inequalities in Health* (Ministry of Health 2002) where it is explained with examples to illustrate its use, and as part of a broader discussion about health inequalities in New Zealand and action needed to address them.

The Intervention Framework was developed particularly for the health sector, although it can be used by any sector concerned with health. Local government, for example, may find it useful in connection with the requirement in the Local Government Act 2002 to use a sustainable development approach to 'promote the social, economic, environmental, and cultural well-being of communities, in the present and for the future'. The framework challenges the health sector to consider its role in the structural pathways that cause inequalities in health, while acknowledging that issues at this level are often not directly within the control of the sector. It argues that the health sector should be an advocate for policies that contribute positively to the determinants of health and reduce inequalities, work collaboratively with other sectors, and use health impact assessment (HIA)[3] (Signal & Durham 2000). HIA has gained some momentum in this country through New Zealand HIA guidelines and training that emphasise Treaty-based and equity-focused HIA (Public Health Advisory Committee 2005).

The framework also focuses on the health sector's role in the intermediary pathways that cause inequalities in health. This role can be both direct, as in community development and health protection, and indirect, as in housing initiatives and local authority policies. In addition, there is some focus on the health sector's role in contributing to, and maintaining, health inequalities through providing equal access to services, improving pathways through care, and taking a population health approach. Lastly, it identifies the ability of the sector to contribute to minimising the impact of disability and illness on socio-economic position, and ultimately on access to all determinants of health.

## The HEAT tool

The Health Equity Assessment Tool (HEAT tool) was developed by the author and other academics at the Wellington School of Medicine and Health Sciences (WSMHS), in partnership with the MoH (Ministry of Health *et al*. 2004) (see Figure 13.2 for the 12 questions of the HEAT tool). Its purpose is to assist users in assessing how particular inequalities in health have developed and to identify intervention points where these inequalities can be tackled effectively. It provides people who are aware of inequalities in health, and willing to address them, with a way to structure their thinking.

The 12-question HEAT tool enables rapid assessment of health policy, services or programmes for their current or future impact on health equity. The simple set of questions challenges users to think more broadly about the equity impacts of health issues and responses. Ideally, it would be used throughout the policy, service, and programme planning process from initial issue identification, through design and implementation, to evaluation of effectiveness. The initial simplicity of the tool may disguise the need for information and research to assist in answering the questions, information that may not always be to hand. The tool is best used by a group of people who reflect the range of views of the community being worked with. Depending on the issue under consideration, the community may be representative of all the people in a region, or they may represent a particular group. If the issue is the provision of accident and emergency services, then the needs of all users of the service will need to be considered, including

---

1. What health issue is the policy/programme trying to address?
2. What inequalities exist in this health area?
3. Who is most advantaged and how?
4. How did the inequality occur? (What are the mechanisms by which this inequality was created, is maintained or increased?)
5. What are the determinants of this inequality?
6. How will you address the Treaty of Waitangi in the context of the New Zealand Public Health and Disability Act 2000?
7. Where/how will you intervene to tackle this issue? Use the Ministry of Health Intervention Framework to guide your thinking.
8. How could this intervention affect health inequalities?
9. Who will benefit most?
10. What might the unintended consequences be?
11. What will you do to make sure it does reduce/eliminate inequalities?
12. How will you know if inequalities have been reduced/eliminated?

---

*Figure 13.2: Questions in Health Equity Assessment Tool for Tackling Inequalities in Health (HEAT Tool) (May 2004). Adapted from Bro Taf Authority 2000 in Ministry of Health, Public Health Consultancy et al. 2004.*

Māori, Pacific, and low-income users. If it is a 'by Māori for Māori' service, the involvement of Māori will be critical to its success. Likewise, if it is a service for young people, the involvement of young people with a range of views will be critical to its success.

The HEAT tool was adapted from part of an HIA tool developed in Wales (Bro Taf Authority 2000) and has been modified in the following ways. The focus of the tool is on who is advantaged – on who is privileged – rather than on the 'victims' of inequity. Focusing on the 'victims' runs the risk of locating the origin of inequity in the purported deficits and failings of individuals rather than with the social institutions and practices that had caused the inequity (Ryan 1971; Lykes *et al.* 1996). For example, Question 3 asks *Who is most advantaged and how?* It explores how inequalities have occurred and what needs to change in order for them to be addressed. Question 6 asks how the initiative will address the Treaty of Waitangi. Taking account of the Treaty is a requirement of the legislation governing the New Zealand health sector, the New Zealand Public Health and Disability Act 2000, and a fundamental principle of the New Zealand Health Strategy (Ministry of Health 2000). The Intervention Framework was included in Question 7 in order to encourage users to take a comprehensive approach to intervention.[4]

The primary use of both tools is to improve the ability of mainstream health policies, services, and programmes to address health inequalities. The focus is not on targeted services that have been established specifically to meet the needs of the most vulnerable in our society because, in fulfilling their mandate, these services are making an important contribution to the task of reducing inequalities in health. Nevertheless, such services may find the tools of value. The tools can be used to consider the equity issues involved in both existing and new policies, services, and programmes, although it is hoped that increasingly all existing health sector policies and interventions will have been scrutinised for equity concerns.

Tools such as these are rare internationally. One such tool, Four Steps Towards Equity, is a health promotion equity tool developed in New South Wales, Australia (South East Health 2003). Like the HEAT tool, it focuses on building equity considerations throughout the planning cycle. It also considers equity principles, organisational capacity, and further supports such as equity websites and key readings.

## Who uses the tools?

District Health Boards manage the largest part of the New Zealand health budget and play a key role in the delivery of hospital and health services. They have a statutory responsibility for reducing health inequalities under the New Zealand Public Health and Disability Act 2000. All DHBs have been required to report on progress in implementing the Intervention Framework in their quarterly reporting on their annual plans since the 2003/4 financial year, and the HEAT tool since 2004/5.

MoH staff are also encouraged to use the tools, which are included in the Ministry of Health Policy Wheel, the framework for the ministry's policy analysis. Staff attending policy analyst training are taught how to use the tools and strongly encouraged to do so.

In addition, the tools have been promoted at forums such as the Public Health Association conference and the first Agencies for Nutrition Action conference on nutrition and physical activity. Other health agencies such as the National Heart Foundation and the Cancer Society have received training in their use. Anecdotal evidence from key contacts concerned with addressing inequalities indicates that the tools have also been used by the National Heart Foundation and Sport and Recreation New Zealand.

## Tools training

Training in the use of the health equity tools was provided as part of a series of sector-wide workshops conducted by Wellington School of Medicine and Health Sciences (WSMHS) in partnership with the MoH in 2003/4 and 2004/5. The purpose of the workshops, 'Tackling inequalities: moving theory to action', was 'to increase the knowledge and skills of District Health Board (DHB) and MoH staff to act on, and advocate for, eliminating inequalities in health in Aotearoa New Zealand'. Approximately 300 staff from the MoH and DHBs as well as members of DHBs participated, including a significant number of senior managers. Further detail about the workshops can be found in the workshop report (Carroll et al. 2004).

The workshops were developed as part of an innovative partnership between academics in the Department of Public Health at the WSMHS and the Reducing Inequalities Policy Team of the MoH. They were based on a needs assessment with senior staff in the MoH and DHBs, who indicated strong support for awareness-raising workshops. Practical, evidence based, and action oriented, the workshops took the social approach to health inequalities outlined earlier in this chapter.

A key focus was to explain the need for an 'equity lens' (Signal 2002). This concept refers to a metaphorical pair of glasses that ensures people ask 'who will benefit' from health sector policies and interventions. It can be used prospectively to assess planned work, or it can be used to critically analyse current services. Without assessing the impact of 'business-as-usual' on existing inequalities, health services run the risk of perpetuating, or even increasing, existing health inequalities (Ministry of Health 2002).

The training programme used ethnic inequalities as a case study, as it is a critical area of widening inequalities in New Zealand and addressing it is consistent with a Treaty of Waitangi approach. This led to a focus on racism as a key driver of ethnic inequalities. The training team used the work of Jones (Jones 1999, 2000), who has developed a framework for understanding racism on three levels – institutionalised, personally mediated, and internalised – and has applied it to health. She argues that this framework is useful for raising new hypotheses about the basis of race-associated differences in health outcomes, as well as for designing effective interventions to eliminate those differences (Jones 2000).

Jones defines institutionalised racism as:

differential access to the goods, services, and opportunities of society by race ... it is structural, having been codified in our institutions of custom, practice, and law, so there need not be an identifiable perpetrator. Indeed, institutionalised racism is often evident as inaction in the face of need (Jones 2000).

Institutional theory was used to understand how health institutions create and maintain inequalities in health (March & Olsen 1984). Proponents of this theory from political science, sociology, and economics argue that 'institutions matter'; that institutions structure the development and implementation of policy, and therefore the programmes and services that result. The approach focuses on the dominant ideas built into institutions, their organisational structures, and the processes and rules by which institutions operate. In the workshops, institutional theory provided a framework for participants not only to analyse how the MoH and DHBs contribute to creating and maintaining inequalities in health, but also to develop action plans to tackle health inequalities through their institutions.

The HEAT tool was used to frame the entire workshop. The initial focus was on existing inequalities and how they occurred, and then moved on to understanding interventions, and evaluating their effectiveness. At each stage in the workshop, the questions in the tool (see Figure 13.2) were applied to the example of heart health. Later, participants had the opportunity to work in small groups and apply the HEAT tool questions to current initiatives in the health sector. Participants often identified an initiative that members of their small group were involved with, such as efforts to reduce obesity, the National Cervical Screening Programme, and the Well Child Tamariki Ora Programme.

Participants rated the workshops highly in their anonymous evaluations and most indicated an increased commitment to tackling inequalities as a result of the training. Key recommendations made to the MoH by the training team at the conclusion of the programme included the critical need for continued sector leadership on the importance of tackling inequalities in health; training for all those who work in the health sector; equity-focused contracting and monitoring frameworks; and the development and dissemination of case studies of efforts to tackle inequalities in health.

## Application and value

In 2004/5 a review was undertaken of the use of the Intervention Framework and the HEAT tool in the New Zealand health sector (Signal & Martin 2005). Methods included an analysis of DHB reporting on efforts to reduce inequalities in health in 2003/4, an analysis of relevant MoH policy documents, an email survey of participants in the training workshops, and focus groups and key informant interviews with MoH and DHB staff members who had knowledge of, or experience with, the tools.

The review found variable use of the tools within both the MoH and the DHBs. They were used and found valuable in some policy areas of the ministry, such as the Family Health Policy Section of the Clinical Services Directorate and in the Public Health Directorate. They were also used in some public health purchasing. In other areas of the ministry, there appeared to be little use of the tools. In terms of use by DHBs, the review noted that all boards were aware of the tools and most used the Intervention Framework in their reporting on inequalities in 2003/4. It appears that the tools are used in many places across the DHBs. However, it was not possible to assess the full extent of their use as only some of the potential users were surveyed or interviewed. Some DHBs reported using the 'intention' of the tools and frameworks rather than applying them at a detailed level. Some incorporated all, or part, of the tools into planning and prioritisation templates, and some reported detailed use of the tools in service reviews. It would appear that those most likely to be using the tools are the funding and planning teams, Māori health teams, primary care teams, and public health units. The majority of DHB informants found the tools useful in their work, particularly in determining priorities for new spending. There are, however, some concerns about the difficulties of applying the tools, or gaining acceptance of them, in the provider arm of DHBs – for example, within hospitals.

The review provided useful information on the strengths and weaknesses of the tools. The HEAT tool is widely viewed as a simple tool that assists users to practise an equity approach in their work. On the other hand, there is a risk that if people are not well informed about equity issues they might not use it appropriately. The Intervention Framework encourages a comprehensive analysis of where to intervene to tackle inequalities in health, but is viewed by some respondents as conceptually challenging; indeed many DHBs had difficulty in assigning their inequalities initiatives to an appropriate level within the tool. The framework's focus on both improving health and reducing inequalities means that interventions to improve health at each of the four levels may not necessarily reduce inequalities as well. Using the Intervention Framework within the HEAT tool (see Figure 8.2, Question 7) reduces this risk, because of the HEAT tool's specific focus on inequalities.

Respondents also identified a limited number of other tools they use to assist them in tackling inequalities, such as the national prioritisation framework, TUHA-NZ (a tool for applying the Treaty in health promotion practice) (Martin 2002), and He Korowai Oranga: Māori Health Strategy, which identifies Māori health and disability priorities (Ministry of Health 2002). Issues identified in the review led to ongoing modification of the tools. The MoH has commissioned the development of a HEAT tool guide and it is due for release in 2007.

## Conclusion

The Intervention Framework and the HEAT tool have a valuable role to play in the critical and challenging enterprise of reducing inequalities in health. Neither, however, is a magic bullet. Ongoing leadership of efforts to tackle inequalities in general is clearly needed, as well as specific leadership in the use of equity tools. The health sector would benefit from the development of, training in, and wider use of other equity tools. The sector would also benefit from a refinement of the Intervention Framework and the HEAT tool and the development of supports to encourage their greater use.

# Part Four
## Intervention Experiences

# 14. The Otara Health story

Olivia James

Poverty and health needs can be portrayed and analysed by statistics and graphs, but working in an area well known for its social and economic deprivation is to be confronted daily with the human reality of the statistics. My 30-year association with the Otara community, and my role in the establishment and management of Otara Health Incorporated, a locally based health promotion organisation, has provided me with insights into the lives of many of Otara's families. My telling of the Otara Health story is therefore both a personal narrative and a history.

## The Otara Community

Otara, the smallest urban ward of Manukau City, has a population of 35,049. However, its ability to hit the headlines, usually with accounts of criminal activity, means that for the many New Zealanders who are unacquainted with this high profile multicultural community, Otara has become a metaphor for the darker side of suburban life.

In the early 1950s, the South Auckland area was expanding and Otara was created as result of central government policy to provide low-cost housing for workers there. Māori, who for generations had lived in inner Auckland city suburbs, were relocated to Otara and were joined by immigrants from the Pacific islands. At this time Māori had no supportive iwi structure, as the area is Tainui and most Māori residents are of Ngapuhi descent. The pan-tribal Otara pioneers designated themselves Ngati Otara. Pacific peoples, similarly, were far away from their island roots and struggling to maintain their separate cultural identities. Initially, Māori was the predominant ethnic group but each census reveals an increase in the numbers of Pacific people and a corresponding proportional decrease in the Māori population. The 2001 Census records 63 per cent Pacific peoples and 21 per cent Māori. Asian, European, and 'other' make up the balance. Half a century after Otara was created, intermarriage has strengthened the concept of Ngati Otara. Health funding in particular – often streamed into artificial silos of Māori, Pacific, and 'mainstream' – has little relevance in this community, which takes the view that we are all in this together.

Rental dwellings account for almost half of Otara's housing stock (44 per cent, Statistics New Zealand website 2001), the majority being owned by Housing New Zealand Corporation (HNZC). The transient nature of some of the tenant families has an ongoing impact on their health, welfare, and education. Although HNZC changes in tenancies have decreased significantly with the introduction of income-related rents in December 2000, the configuration of households changes frequently. Young people introduce their partners, babies join the *aiga* or whānau, and overseas relatives stay for extended visits.

HNZC's Healthy Housing programme, a partnership with Counties Manukau District Health Board (CMDHB), was introduced in 2000, with the aim of reducing meningococcal disease and enhancing health outcomes through the modification and extension of homes, health education, and improved linkages to local health services. The Healthy Housing programme has been a positive influence in lifting the standard of housing in the ward and mitigating some of the worst overcrowding. Nevertheless, overcrowding is still an issue as a determinant of poor health.

There is a dichotomy to Otara: on the one hand there are the minority whose life stories are akin to those of the characters in *Once Were Warriors*,[1] and on the other, the mature and visionary leadership, the multicultural taonga of Otara. In between these two extremes are the many thousands of families represented in the stark statistics which spell out poverty and health needs in Aotearoa.

The hardship experienced on a day-to-day basis by many families is demonstrated in the following excerpts from *Discounting Health and Healthcare in Low Income Households in Otara* (Cheer 2000: 109).

> The amount of money we have for food changes each week depending on what cultural occasions come up. If there's none there is more money for food. If there's many then it is back to bread and jam. Last week there was only $30 for food because there was a funeral to pay for … Ideally it would take about $150 to feed everyone well, but even on weeks when there's no cultural things we still don't have that much …

> My boy's shoe in front is talking to him. The sole has come off and whenever he walks it slaps on the ground and talks to him. I had to get him new shoes so I had to stop the automatic payments that week (power and telephone). I couldn't use lay-by because he needed the shoes straight away. And then I got charged by the bank for changing the AP. (Cheer 2000: 117)

> One day the kids were really hungry and we just didn't have any food. They went to Ioana's house and knocked on the door 'Ioana, can we have some food.' She had some left over potatoes in the pot and gave them to the kids even though her son hadn't eaten yet. He had no potatoes that night just so my kids could have something to eat. (Cheer 2000: 118)

Sometimes Dad and I will have to not eat so that the kids have enough. We'll just have bread and a cup of tea instead. But sometimes there's not even enough to feed the kids. (Cheer 2000: 124)

The house affects our health a hell of a lot. Water seeps into the house, there's damp windowsills, rotting wood and it gets really cold. (Cheer 2000: 130)

The story of the establishment and ongoing viability of Otara Health Incorporated is a tribute to the spirit of this unique community and touches upon what is required to address its needs.

## Establishment processes

From the start, the poor health of the Otara community was very visible to both residents and health professionals. The onset of diseases was accepted with resignation, and the presence of residents in their seventies and beyond was a rarity. It was widely accepted that every baby born in Otara had a 50 per cent chance of being hospitalised before its first birthday.

In early 1994 a group of community leaders and health professionals began meeting. They sought a solution to this parlous state of affairs. After careful debate, the proposal for a one-stop shop, incorporating health and welfare agencies, information services, and possibly an overnight short-stay facility was developed. The Northern Regional Health Authority (North Health) declined the group's submission, observing quite accurately that they funded services not bricks and mortar. The story may well have ended there except for the resolve of the group and the persistence of a Manukau City Councillor, Len Brown, who took up the cause on behalf of his Otara community. North Health's governance was reminded of its mission 'Bringing health care as close as possible to where people live and work' (North Health 1995). An Otara health needs analysis was commissioned (Mitchell 1995) and oversight of the initiative was handed to North Health's Pacific team, presumably in recognition of Otara's demography. Three years' persistence paid off, and in 1997 the local working group was directed to form a legal entity with which North Health could contract. Otara Health was incorporated on 13 October 1997.

The favoured form of primary health service delivery postulated at the time was Co-ordinating Care Organisations (CCOs). The CCO strategy is described in a North Health discussion document:

In summary, your primary care provider is the person(s) you turn to first for advice, information, help with deciding what to do and how to do it, basic treatment and help with accessing specialised services. Your primary care provider will also assist you in co-ordinating the various services you need to produce the best results for you. This person may well be a general practitioner but is not necessarily so. Many different professionals are involved including pharmacists, nurses and community health workers (North Health 1995).

An 'Agreement for the Establishment of Co-ordinated Care Services' was signed between Otara Health Inc. and the Health Funding Authority as the purchaser of Health and Disability Services for the people in the North Region on 12 March 1998.

It is fair to say that the North Health bureaucracy was not enthusiastic. After all, an organisation that was community based and driven, fitting neither Māori, Pacific, nor mainstream moulds, did not match with the usual organisational criteria. The hope was implied, although not expressed, that this camel designed by a committee would, after a minimum period of time, quietly slink away never to be seen again.

The CCO strategy, which did not find favour with the medical professions, was shortlived, but the foundation principles are seen today in the New Zealand Health Strategy and the Primary Health Organisations (PHOs) which deliver the services. The inconsistency of working to a CCO agreement when CCOs were non-existent was to be a challenge over the next seven years. It is to the credit of the five funding bodies (North Health, Transitional Health Funding Authority, Regional Health Funding Authority, Health Funding Authority, and Counties Manukau District Health Board), with whom Otara Health Incorporated did business over the next five years of ongoing health 'reforms', that they allowed the organisation to develop according to its response to community needs rather than enforcing the fine print of the service agreement.

# Beginnings

If the Otara Health Inc. venture was to succeed, community buy-in was essential. The new organisation had to be seen to be providing an acceptable and visible response to community health needs. The diversity of Otara's communities needed to be represented in its governance, with strong community leadership blended with health professional expertise. These matters were a priority. Equally pressing were the practical details of identifying suitable and affordable premises and staff recruitment.

## Community engagement

The Otara Primary and Public Needs Assessment Report (an in-house report for the period 1995-6 initiated by the Auckland Regional Health Authority) had identified that there was no shortage of services available to Otara. Community uptake was another thing. Common barriers to the utilisation of available services were cost, transport, and language. Thirty equally valid but less overt barriers to care were identified by Dr David Simmons in a major study undertaken in inner urban South Auckland (Simmons et al. 1998).

Clearly, traversing the bridge between accessible health services and the will to utilise those services was too hard for many. The obvious answer lay in providing help to cross the bridge, to smooth the way. 'Way-smoothers' (and Otara Health has yet to find a more appropriate term) became the standard and accepted means of bringing help, support, information, and confidence to the people. The titles of the way-smoothers are many depending on their role – community health workers, ambassadors, activity champions – but the core function is similar. Staff at Otara Health, including the way-smoothers, are, in the main, Otara or Manukau City residents, and most are multilingual. They relate to people on a platform of equality and make the inaccessible accessible.

The way-smoother philosophy is interwoven into all aspects of the services provided by Otara Health, and is an integral part of its founding principles. These include real community involvement at all levels; a multilingual workforce drawn from the local community; intersectoral collaboration; health education provided on a one-to-one basis or in small interactive groups; responsiveness to feedback; projects developed on the basis of community need; and transparent and accountable business and financial systems.

## Governance

If community buy-in was important at an operational level, it was equally as important in the organisation's governance. It was important that all parties were fairly represented on the board because this venture was, in theory at any rate, a partnership between the health sector and the community. The organisation's constitution, 'The Rules of Otara Health Inc.', provides for equal numbers of Otara health professionals and community representatives drawn from the predominant ethnic groups. Each representative is appointed annually by their constituent group.

Early community meetings, called to decide on the representatives, were spirited affairs. There were high expectations of performance, consultation, and feedback. Representatives who did not shape up were summarily replaced the following year. Community scrutiny of their representatives has become more relaxed over recent years, with acceptance of the organisation's role and the direct benefits many families have experienced from programmes initiated by Otara Health.

With the common goal of enacting the Mission Statement 'Creating Good Health For Otara People', the mix of professional and lay people melded together surprisingly quickly. The health providers valued genuine unadorned community feedback, and the community people learned that health service delivery was not a straightforward business, particularly in a climate of constant 'reform'.

The value-base of the Otara Health Inc. board, in respect of its community development principles, is exemplified in these excerpts from a 'Belief Statement':

We believe that a community has the right to choose the direction of its own development.

We believe that the community people know their problems and the solutions that will work better than others know them.

We believe that there are resources and skills within each community that are under-utilised waiting to be harnessed.

We believe that the main actors that make the plans and work the action should be the people with the problem. (Community Forum 1997)

## Intersectoral Cooperation and Support

The support of the local authority, Manukau City Council, has been a significant factor in the establishment and ongoing operation of Otara Health. The organisation's main office is in council-owned premises in the heart of the Otara shopping centre, adjacent to the Citizens Advice Bureau and other community and social service agencies. Initially a commercial rental was paid, but this was substantially reduced in 2001 with the introduction of the council's community tenancy policy. Two grants from the council's social development fund, each of $30,000 in years one and two, were a great help in setting up the office and employing the three staff – a manager, a community worker, and an administrator. Intersectoral cooperation and support was to become an invaluable factor in service development as Otara Health increasingly became involved in programmes addressing the determinants of health. Funding through the CCO agreement took care of the infrastructure and overheads, but did not allow for any significant project development. As previously indicated, the concept of CCOs, as foreshadowed in North Health's strategy, was not viable. As the first manager of Otara Health, Ian McKenzie reflected, coordinating organisations which have no intention of being coordinated is akin to herding feral cats. The pragmatic way ahead was to identify gaps in service delivery, to develop programmes that would add value to existing services, and to include Otara residents in the action. Funding had to be found, but because Otara Health was neither a Māori nor a Pacific organisation (despite 84 per cent of its constituencies being of these ethnicities) health funding for specific projects was always declined. Working with organisations whose criteria were less rigid became a necessity.

From the outset it was agreed that volunteer labour was not an option. Both the board and staff of Otara Health held the view that local knowledge, practical skills, and multilingual ability were assets that should be paid for. Everyone working for the organisation, whether on a permanent basis or on a short-term project, had a formal employment agreement including a commitment to upskilling and ongoing training. The hourly rate paid was never less than $12 (at a time when the minimum wage was $7), more if expected outcomes were particularly demanding and the budget could be stretched. This expectation of professionalism paid big dividends in human terms.

A number of projects were funded through the Work and Income (W&I) Task Force Green Scheme, for people who had been unemployed for three years or more. Around 75 per cent of people who have worked on short-term projects for Otara Health have moved on to permanent paid employment. The benefits of increased self-esteem and pride in the organisation and the community are inestimable.

## Meningococcal and TB awareness

Two early Otara Health projects forged a productive and congenial working relationship with the Auckland Regional Public Health Service (ARPHS). These were participation in a meningococcal awareness programme and support for a mass Mantoux testing[2] programme at a local college.

The meningococcal awareness-raising programme was initiated by Auckland Healthcare and involved a team of six local people, through a W&I employment scheme, providing information door to door. Otara Health was not happy with the coverage achieved and took responsibility for extending the scheme to ensure at least 90 per cent coverage. Similar awareness programmes were undertaken each year until the meningococcal vaccination programme was launched in 2004. The simple message of getting suspicious symptoms checked out immediately had a definite impact. Although the incidence of the disease remained constant in Otara, anecdotal reports from Middlemore Hospital staff indicated that they were seeing patients earlier than those from more affluent South Auckland suburbs that had not had the benefit of a one-to-one awareness-raising programme.

Just as the 1998 meningococcal awareness programme was finishing, banner headlines on the front page of the *New Zealand Herald* (3 September) announced an outbreak of tuberculosis at Tangaroa College, one of Otara's two secondary schools. Otara Health's offer of assistance to ARPHS was politely declined. Public health nurses were dealing with the situation, administering Mantoux tests, and following up families. Ten days later an anxious ARPHS reported that parents were not signing consent forms and the testing had stalled. Could Otara Health help? The meningococcal awareness team, after a half-day orientation and briefing on the purpose of the Mantoux, swung into action talking to parents, alleviating their fears, and leaving homes with signed consents. Only six families refused. This was a concrete example of the value of the 'way-smoother' approach.

Directly Observed Therapy (DOT), personally administering medication to non-compliant TB patients, had always been undertaken by public health nurses. This was proving to be a time-consuming and expensive exercise. ARPHS had been considering employing trained lay people. Following the Tangaroa College incident, it was suggested that a collaborative pilot should be trialled, with ARPHS providing training and clinical oversight and Otara Health being the employing and administrative body. The outcome was successful and non-clinical DOT workers are now directly employed by ARPHS. The ability of one Samoan worker, who took part in the pilot and was then employed by Otara Health, is legendary, particularly among her own community.

# Health-related housing projects

The National Health Committee report, *The Social, Cultural and Economic Determinants of Health in New Zealand: Action to Improve Health* (1998), highlighted the connection between health and housing and recommended a number of changes. The Minister of Health at that time described the report's findings as 'old news' and called for more work on 'local solutions for local problems'. This challenge was taken up by Dr Chris Bullen of ARPHS, who invited a group of Otara community leaders and agency representatives to consider the minister's response. Participants were well aware that government decisions on social and economic policy determined the reality of their circumstances, but nevertheless were open to considering local solutions for local problems. This project became known as the Otara Housing and Health Local Solutions Project. The outcomes and recommendations were to have considerable influence on Otara Health's direction over the following two years.

The Bullen report to the National Health Committee, which funded the project, made a number of recommendations to statutory agencies servicing Otara. Two other proposals for action were taken up by Otara Health: a healthy housing education and information campaign (the Otara Health and Housing Campaign) and research on housing design (*Our Home, Our Place*). (A third proposal described research on how families on low incomes in Otara survive despite relatively high rentals (Cheer 2000; Cheer *et al.* 2002)). The Otara Health and Housing Campaign and *Our Home, Our Place* led to further housing projects such as Otara's participation in the University of Otago's Housing, Insulation and Health Study (HIHS), and the groundbreaking HNZC Healthy Housing initiative.

## *Otara Health and Housing Campaign*

The Otara Health and Housing Campaign (known as the Ambassadors Project) was a programme initiated and coordinated by Otara Health, but dependent on inter-agency cooperation and funding. Participating agencies were Manukau City Council, Housing New Zealand, Work and Income, and the New Zealand Fire Service. Nine bilingual 'ambassadors' were selected from local long-term unemployed people, who were then trained on issues relating to public health, fire prevention, house maintenance, and benefit entitlements.

> The Ambassadors visited a total of 7191 houses, carried out 2200 interviews (31 per cent) and gave written information only to 2494 households (35 per cent). The remaining households (34 per cent) were not contacted for a variety of reasons such as locked gates, dogs, house empty and advice not wanted. Ambassadors dealt with 299 rat/mice infestations and made 481 referrals to official agencies regarding house maintenance, benefits and health issues. (Haigh 2000)

The Ambassadors Project raised the profile of Otara Health on many levels.

The community experienced real improvements in their living environment as a result of the ambassadors' interventions, while statutory agencies involved in the project experienced the benefits of interaction with each other and the communities they served. 'It was really a "Whole of Government" approach and we were doing it in Otara years before anywhere else' (Denise Wiki, HNZC, pers. comm., August 2004).

The project was repeated in 2002, again with positive community outcomes. As a result Manukau City Council initiated a three-year contract with Otara Health to provide environmental education to the Otara ward of the city.

### Our Home, Our Place

*Our Home, Our Place* identified many examples of common housing design that are incompatible with cultural beliefs and practices. Otara Health convened a Housing Reference Group. For some time the group had considered the fact that most of Otara's housing was built for small nuclear families (the parents and three children), rather than the extended Māori and Pacific families who actually occupied them. The group also believed that many aspects of the design of these houses did not cater for the cultural and physical needs of the people who were living in them.

For example, design inadequacy becomes obvious when, after the death of a family member, the body is brought home to lie in state prior to burial. Standard low-cost design means that it is impossible for a coffin to be brought through the front door into the passage and then turned to gain entry to the sitting room. The only solution is to break the window of the sitting room to allow access for the coffin. This means temporary coverage for the broken window and eventually the cost of replacing the glass. (The generosity of spirit of Otara people means that a number of Pacific people now lie in state on Ngati Otara marae rather than in their home.)

In 2001 the Otara Health and the Housing Reference Group convened a hui, not to share ideas on how the existing housing stock in Otara could be adapted, but rather to develop ideas on how new housing could be radically rethought to move away from the conventional design ideas aimed at middle-class Pakeha households. The interactive process was convened by Rau Hoskins (architect) and Alan Johnson (planner) and resulted in a report identifying concerns, reasons, and emerging themes (Johnson & James 2001). Māori and Pacific people, who made up 90 per cent of the participants, identified housing issues relevant to their cultures. There was remarkable convergence of views and the outcome was the development of a house designed to meet the practical and cultural needs of both groups. The report was widely distributed and was congruent with similar research undertaken elsewhere in the country. The dream of the Housing Reference Group was to have a prototype house built in Otara. HNZC undertook to identify available land and explore funding options. Habitat for Humanity was open to involvement in building the house. Regrettably nothing eventuated.

## Insulation

As mentioned earlier in this chapter, Otara was one of seven communities in Aotearoa to participate in the Housing, Insulation and Health Study (HIHS), a multidisciplinary research programme undertaken by the University of Otago to explore the causal links between living in a warmer house and health improvement. The research extended over a two-year period. Otara Health, the coordinating agency, employed workers to identify uninsulated households in which at least one person had ongoing respiratory problems. Householders were to record their perceptions of warmth as 'warm', 'cold' or 'okay'. Family health status over the three-month winter period of 2001 was monitored and other household information recorded. Half of the houses were insulated in the summvvver of 2001 and the remainder at the completion of the research in summer 2002 (Howden-Chapman *et al.* 2005).

Financial constraints precluded the majority of participants from using any form of heating, but insulation increased the comfort in the home. As one participant in the HIHS anecdotally noted, 'The kids don't wear socks inside anymore ... sometimes it is cold, but it is different, a *dry* cold'.

While the immediate benefits were obvious to Otara Health (200 homes insulated to a high standard, free of charge to the occupant), community people, cautious of yet another research spotlight being focused on Otara, were initially reluctant to become involved. It took the persuasion of a senior Kaumatua to get the numbers. However, once the benefits of insulation became apparent, Otara Health was overwhelmed with demands for their homes to be insulated under the project. Unfortunately, it was too late for many households.

## Housing New Zealand Corporation's programme for healthy housing

Concurrently with the HIHS, HNZC embarked on a programme to insulate all of their housing stock in the region, a positive development in housing improvement in Otara. Regrettably the area's absentee landlords in the private sector have shown little inclination to upgrade their properties, and the ambassadors, community health workers, and visiting health professionals too often found substandard and dangerous living conditions for which market rents are demanded. As the then CEO of HNZC, Michael Lennon, has observed: 'It is worth investigating why leaky buildings, as a housing issue, received so much attention; while the issue of housing poverty has received much less' (Lennon 2003). Otara Health agrees.

HNZC's Healthy Housing programme, initially designed to reduce overcrowding, has evolved to include a comprehensive set of interventions such as insulation, ventilation, internal redesign and maintenance, household education around health risk reduction, and facilitating linkages with health and social support agencies (Housing New Zealand Corporation 2003). As described earlier in this chapter, Otara, one of the three areas in Auckland with the highest rates of meningococcal disease, was a participant in HNZC's Healthy Housing programme.

Otara Health was contracted to support families in Healthy Housing homes by reinforcing the health education work of the public health nurse and making links with available community-based services like Citizens Advice Bureau, Salvation Army, and budgeting services. The worker had some success with encouraging clients to rejoin the work force or retrain. She also demonstrated basic housekeeping techniques ('Don't buy all those expensive cleaners. A capful of bleach in a bucket of water does the trick'). She was watchful that overcrowding did not re-emerge. ('I count the beds!')

## Other Otara Health Programmes

Otara Health provides numerous programmes and services, some based on the determinants of health, others offering health education in a context acceptable to the people it serves. The following are a sample of such initiatives.

### Injury prevention

In a community where many are living on or below the breadline, the cost of a driver's licence or infant car restraint can seem an unaffordable luxury. As a health issue, however, the levels of transport-related injury in Otara could not be ignored. The catalyst was an urgent request from Plunket, whose Otara Infant Car Seat scheme had collapsed: no seats, no money, no volunteers. In a marathon effort, Otara Health raised $65,000 in one month, purchased 100 top-of-the-range seats and invested the balance to ensure that capital for future purchasing would always be available. The Mayor of Manukau, Sir Barry Curtis, added his weight to the fundraising by using his influence to attract corporate donations. As well as being a gesture of his personal goodwill, it reinforced Otara Health's conviction of the value of networking and making intersectoral linkages.

In terms of driver licences, Otara Health has worked with Land Transport New Zealand since 2002 to provide tuition for learner's licences. The tutor is Samoan and delivers the training in that language, when appropriate.

Despite these ongoing efforts, much remains to be achieved in terms of injury protection in a low-income community where costs of rent, debt servicing, food, clothing, and transport make the saving of even small sums for such safeguards yet another financial burden.

### Women's health

A series of workshops was undertaken by Otara Health in partnership with the Salvation Army with the objective of opening up the taboo subjects of sex education, contraception, homosexuality, and so on. The need for such open discussion was highlighted by a conversation with the Director of the Family Planning Association, who cited the case of a Pacific Island woman who had just had her seventh abortion. This worthwhile workshop project had to be discontinued because of insufficient funding.

*Traditional healers*

The role of the *fofo*, or traditional healer, in Otara is significant. For two years Otara Health attempted, unsuccessfully, to create a climate where the healer and the general practitioner were able to work collegially in the best interests of the patient. The gap was too wide and no significant gains were achieved. Middlemore Hospital has since approved a traditional healing policy, and other health agencies are investigating the importance of traditional healing in multicultural communities.

*Public presentations*

Otara Health coordinates promotions such as Well Child Week and Diabetes Awareness Week in the Otara Town Centre, the hub of the community. While such events are always enthusiastically received and provide excellent opportunities for inter-agency networking, it is Otara Health's view that posters and slogans do not change behaviours, whereas sustained support and one-to-one interaction are more likely to achieve a positive result.

# PHO – Total Healthcare Otara

Otara Health has continued to evolve as opportunities have arisen. It welcomed the introduction of the New Zealand Health Strategy announced in December 2000, as the principles were congruent with Otara Health's values and its practice of working collaboratively with the community and a range of health and welfare service providers.

The Primary Health Care Strategy (February 2001) signalled the formation of Primary Health Organisations (PHOs) as a means of implementing the strategy. It was Otara Health's hope that one Otara PHO would be established; however, differing philosophical attitudes among local health providers made this impracticable. The ongoing challenge is to develop and maintain practical working relationships with Otara's four PHOs. Good progress has been made in the health promotion area.

On 1 January 2003 Otara Health joined East Tamaki Healthcare, the biggest provider of general practice services in Otara (enrolled population 74,000), to form the PHO Total Healthcare Otara. Otara Health maintained its autonomy as an independent provider of health promotion services to the community and works under a provider agreement employing 11 community health workers who between them speak seven languages and several Hindi dialects. They are competent, trained people who provide one-to one-health education and disease management information as well as case-managing referrals to social agencies and disability support services.

PHO funding also enabled Otara Health to employ a health promotion team with the financial resources to develop and implement some innovative community-based programmes. One of the most successful is 'Getting Started', a partnership between Otara Health, Manukau City Council, and the

Sport and Recreation Council (SPARC). Doctors refer their patients to Otara Health. They are then contacted by an activity champion, who explains the programme and accompanies them on their first visit to the Leisure Centre, introducing them to the staff, who develop a personalised fitness programme for them. The activity champion is present at all 'Getting Started' programmes, providing encouragement and support. Nutrition sessions are realistically geared to accommodate restricted budgets. The inclusive and supportive nature of 'Getting Started' means that friends and whānau are also attracted to join. Although the programme is expensive and labour intensive, it is money well spent because it works.

## Conclusion

Otara Health started with three staff and an uncertain one-year contract. Seven years later an enthusiastic staff of 25, mostly local people, were doing the mahi. In the background, a small team of professional people support the community process, help with the development of ideas, set up systems, and monitor accountabilities, guided by the principles on which it was founded, and those of Ottawa Charter for Health Promotion (World Health Organization 1986), in particular to build healthy public policy, create supportive environments, strengthen community action, develop personal skills, and re-orient health services.

The way-smoother philosophy is interwoven into all aspects of the services provided by Otara Health Inc., and is an integral part of the principles on which Otara Health was founded. These include real community involvement at all levels; a multilingual workforce drawn from the local community; intersectoral collaboration; health education provided one-to-one or in small interactive groups; responsiveness to feedback and projects developed on the basis of community need; and transparent and accountable business and financial systems.

While health inequalities and need are demonstrated daily, the Otara Health story shows that a community labelled as disadvantaged can effectively provide local solutions to local problems.

# 15. Stories from people working with high needs populations

Win Bennett, Eugene Ryder, Maude Governor,
Kathy James, Maggie Simcox, and Lianne Ormsby

The reflections and stories in this chapter come from people working to improve the health of people with high needs. They were recorded at a symposium on health inequalities in 2004,[1] and were provided by a number of speakers working in different but related ways with people at the coalface. The speakers, all from the Wellington area, were Eugene Ryder, Maude Governor, and Kathy James from the Newtown Union Health Service; Maggie Simcox, a practice nurse at Waitangirua; and Lianne Ormsby from the Maraeroa Marae Clinic. The chapter highlights some common issues and themes that a number of these stories touched upon, as well as the importance of establishing relationships through empathy, patience, and teamwork in order to be effective in this environment.

One of the dominant threads that run through the stories is that many people with high health needs do not feel part of or able to approach the usual health services. The failure of these services to be welcoming to and accepting of the people in the following stories will probably be surprising, and even alarming, to many people working in more mainstream health care systems.[2] These stories have been collected by those who are 'working in the gap' – the gap between those who need health services and those who deliver them in mainstream ways. They illuminate how some groups and individuals outside the mainstream see these services.

Eugene Ryder, a community health worker for Nga Mokai Whānau Ora, vividly describes the perspective of some gang members:

> A few of the boys, they look at the medical institution the same way they look at prison officers, the same way they look at cops and the same way they look at teachers – some of the boys won't talk to you unless you've got a patch on, they can't relate to you, they don't want to know you. Some of these things that I come across, in some instances it's just ignorance, but that's reality.

Lianne Ormsby has a long history of working in the health services:

> I've worked in, as a midwife, Wellington Hospital for 16 years and I thought I was doing really a great job there. I fixed them all up and send them all off home thinking well that's it I've done a good job and it wasn't actually until I

got to Porirua, I've been out in the community now for six years, and realised that I was actually sending them home to cold houses, this was mothers and babies … no food in their cupboards. We give these young girls scrips to go home for blood pressures and they have no money to even go and get their pills from the chemist.

So since I've been out there I have just suddenly realised that: why was I even in the hospital, I should have been out in the community ages ago… I mean I see all those things, houses with mould on, cold houses … I actually do the Tamariki Hauora contract too for the clinic and I go into houses to weigh babies and I go in and I've got a coat on and we take our shoes off and it's just so cold and they say… oh, you've come to weigh the baby and we say, oh yes, we'll weigh the baby but I have had to estimate how much the clothes are going to weigh because I'm too scared to take all the clothes off because it's so cold. So, I'm amazed sometimes how some of our babies survive out there but we might fix that up sometime.

Lianne goes on to tell a story that shows the perspective of an older Maori man:

We were having a Diabetic Support Group clinic and one of the ladies came up to me and said, can you go and have a look at my cousin, his legs are all weird and swollen and he won't go and see the doctor. I had a look at his legs and they were red and he had some cream and I said I'd put some on – that was all he was willing for me to do at the time. I asked him how his diabetes was and he said it has got nothing to do with you, so I said okay then I'll say no more … I went back twice a week to go and put cream on his legs and over a period of time he said, so where are you from Lianne … so we started talking about iwi and other people and so I snuck in a little bit about diabetes and he said, 'Oh, it's fine, it's fine.' And then as we went on, his legs actually got worse and I said maybe we should go to the doctor, and he said, 'Oh I go to the doctor and he don't do nothing.'

Maggie Simcox tells of a Pacific Island woman who, for a long time, had been afraid of the hospital:

… and finally she admitted to me that she had this lump in her groin and it became evident she believed it was cancer and she'd had it for seven years and because of it she and her husband had had no intimacy, so no sexual relationship for seven years because of this lump. She was terrified it was cancer and again slowly she let me have a look. It didn't look like a cancer. And again, it seemed, her face softened – but with the mention of the hospital, fear again. For many of our patients, hospital is a place where you only go in one direction and you don't come out. So there is a huge amount of fear with that.

But this failure in service delivery can be changed, and an important dimension of this change is the establishment of relationships. Eugene notes:

A lot of the work that I do is in the part of the community that is proportionately small and that is represented highly in all the negative statistics that are out there. I thought I'd give a talk on what works with the community that I'm representing and basically whatever works, works ... Basically I ask the boys what's going to get you there bro, you know, and some of them might need a ride, some of them might need money, just whatever it takes to get them there. I think one of the keys to the success of a lot of the workers at the coalface is the relationship they have with their clients. I was lucky, I am part of the people that I'm working with, and that's what works. When I was young, people were telling me what to do and what was right and wrong, and they learnt that from a book, so I ignored everything they said, which cost me a few years in jail, but from that I've learnt that it's those experiences that help me relate to what they're talking about. They know you've been there and they know what you've been through, and that you know what they're about to go through. So that's part of the healing process.

Maude Governor also reflects on what helps her establish meaningful and effective relationships:

What do I do that makes a difference? Simply being Maori makes all the difference. Being proud of who I am and who I represent. I bring to this role not just my strengths, but the strengths, gifts, and talents of my Whanau, Iwi and Tipuna.

Maude then describes what she is passionate about:

My ... story is about the Maori diabetes roopu (group). The roopu was established to identify the needs and priorities of our Maori diabetes members, and to put in place an action plan that would address those needs. As a result, we have held a number of sessions on diabetes education, podiatry, sports education, supermarket tours, and health promotion hui. Regular group exercise of line dancing, aqua jogging, walking, and Tai Chi have all contributed towards improving their health and well-being. We have also established a vegetable garden so that members are able to access fresh vegetables. These sessions have enabled members and their whanau to learn to manage their diabetes and prevent complications through diabetes education, healthy lifestyle changes, and regular exercise.

She also relates the following success story:

The breast-screening project of Maori women from Newtown Union Health Service was a success because the Maori community health worker coordinated it. The breast screening health promoter was Maori. Members knew they were attending the screening as a roopu, to tautoko and awhi (support) each other. The environment was welcoming and they were greeted with aroha, warmth, and affection. Most important of all, they were treated with dignity and respect. As a result of this project Maori women from Newtown Union Health Service accessing breast screening increased from 20 per cent to 80 per cent.

Maggie Simcox describes the importance of patient trust in this piece about the Pacific Island woman who feared going to hospital:

> We were able to get someone on board who was the same [ethnicity]... and could share much more deeply and more intimately with her. She took her to the hospital to see the specialist, the assessment, to the pre-assessment and then for her operation. Again she was still very, very frightened and very reluctant to go and had we not had the access nurse [a nurse working in primary care who coordinates services for people with complex health issues] with us I think it might have been very different. So she did go, she came out after she'd had the operation, it was only, again best medical words, a fatty lump and the outcome from that was fine.

Lianne explains how the older Māori man was able to access health services:

> Then the next thing was we took him to the podiatrist because we hadn't got that far; we'd got him to the doctors so we thought we'd try him with the podiatrist because he had a little cut on his heel. So we got him to the podiatrist and she said she felt he needed to go to the vascular surgeon, so he said, 'What's that, Lianne? And I said, 'Well, they just want to see if there is any blood going down to your feet.' – 'Aw ... okay.' So away we went to the vascular surgeon.
>
> I just want to tell you that ever since he had diabetes he wrote this paper on how he was a diabetic and his dream was that he wanted to do a hikoi [a term that often refers to a long journey or march] from the top of the North Island right down to the bottom of the South Island, going into the marae and talking about his diabetes, and especially to the young. So this was his dream, his hikoi about his diabetes. But then his hip started playing up so he couldn't get any further but when we came in, his dreams all came alive again – so now he wants his hip fixed: so, okay.

Kathy James talks about providing holistic care for patients with complex needs:

> We have got over 32 different languages spoken at Newtown Union Health. Someone described Newtown to me as a mainstream health service working in a bicultural society with a multicultural population. That left me to think ...
>
> On a personal level for patients, the focus is really moving away from crisis and curative services, although that is very important when someone is very

sick to [be able to] access services easily. But we need to pay more attention to managing patients with high and complex health needs, and usually these patients have multiple co-morbidities. Developments of multi-disciplinary teams and shared care arrangements are going to be key to this, alongside the undervalued continuity of care which I think is one of the essential parts of the glue that underpins many of the primary health care strategies.

Her story is about a woman:

She had frequent visits to the clinic, usually in crisis. She would drop in with breathlessness, chest pain, painful joints and it was really very hard to get any traction on managing some of her multiple issues. I sat down with her and the nurse and we had a discussion about how we should proceed and she agreed to come in for regular visits with me once a month and we'd slowly chip away at some of the issues that needed addressing. At the end of the talk about my stuff, which was the medical stuff, I asked her what she liked and she told me that she loved fishing every day at the wharf and the best thing that she wanted was to be able to read and write. So at that meeting we gave her the telephone number for the adult literacy programme and she made some contact with them. I provided regular review, monthly appointments. She saw the asthma nurse. We investigated her ischaemic heart disease and we treated her hypertension and we addressed the issue of binge drinking which had come up in previous consultations. She was really delighted because she had been able to read, at one of her clinic appointments, a children's picture book – she could actually sit there and read, and she was so pleased with that. She had made changes to move away from friends that had been encouraging her into drinking and she had established contact with her family with whom she had had no previous contact over the last 20 years.

Her hypertension was well controlled, she had been started on statin drugs, she developed an asthma plan with the nurse, and she was now self-managing her asthma. She had stopped drinking. She was really pleased because she had been able to fill in and sign her Invalid's Benefit form. Her father had commented to her how well she looked and they were really interested to know what was happening for her in Wellington. That gave her a real buzz because she realised that something was happening for herself that was different. She was very worried that the family were coming down to visit for Christmas and what was going to happen, and over a period of time they negotiated that people would smoke outside her place and they would have a dry Christmas. She commented that she really liked the magazines in the clinic.

She now has regular visits to the GP and the nurse, and these are really about maintenance and she continues to self-manage. She has been reading the newspaper. She has made changes in her personal life and for the first time she has applied for a passport. Her gout flares up sometimes, she is still self-managing her asthma and COPD [Chronic Obstructive Pulmonary Disease], blood pressure is controlled and investigations for her heart disease have been completed. She made her first trip overseas. She can read novels.... She attends Maude's group on healthy eating and she has been to the Tai Chi class.

These stories highlight some important keys to success for these health workers. They also highlight the need for perseverance, the ability to empathise with a patient's history and circumstances, patience, cooperation, and teamwork with colleagues as well as with patients. Two essential skills required by these workers seem to be the ability and willingness to listen and empower. The stories show that a university degree is not necessary – humility and caring are. Maggie Simcox concludes her story by saying:

> It was great to see her and she is doing really well and is happy and confident. So my thing again is we all work together, like the GP, the access nurse, the secondary care, the hospital were good and quick and she got in quickly. I'm a practice nurse and to me that is the only way we are going to work and go forward together.

Lianne:

> Our work in Porirua is what they want, we do everything, but it's actually a team effort, it's not only me who sees them, the community support person sees them, the community health worker sees them, everybody goes there because he's [the older Maori man with swollen legs] our Koro. At the moment he's teaching us Te Reo and Tikanga one hour a week.

Kathy James:

> Health services are about more than going to the doctor. They involve outreach services and suitcase clinics and taking the services out to where people are. Although we have a framework for Primary Health Care in New Zealand, I think we need to ask what really underpins that at a practical level. I call that 'the glue'. What's the glue that makes it work? One of the keys to that is community participation – and that's not only the community being involved in health services, but includes health services being involved with the community. It's a subtle but important difference. Trusting relationships. Building up community trust takes a long time and it can be lost very easily. Respect and understanding of cultural differences.

These stories are of events in an economically rich country with well-organised health, educational, and community services. So if we as a society are committed to reducing health inequalities, what are the implications for policy-makers, researchers, and service managers? First, we need to be aware that inequalities are part of our health environment, and to understand that the dynamics that underlie them are different from those that apply to mainstream services. One size does not fit all, as mainstream services assume. On the contrary, these services do not fit those outside the mainstream, as among these people there is little or no understanding of the service being provided or faith in it. Second, we need to be wary – without understanding, it is easy to make things worse. Listening to people from the communities and those working closely with them, and being alert to unintended consequences of even the most well-intentioned actions is crucial. Third, we should never patronise: there is a rich humanity in all these stories – strength, insight, love and commitment – and sometimes we just need to support with resources and get out of the way. Fourth, we need to be realistic about the depth of resources and the timeframes that are really needed to enable this kind of change. Be generous, have faith, and be humble – the rewards may be great.

Winning hearts may be more important than winning minds. Most of the people in these stories did have access to services, and when they felt comfortable took advantage of them, some becoming advocates for the same services they had initially rejected. Much has been written on defining and describing inequalities: our problem seems to be turning this into effective action.

A further implication in these stories is that policy-makers should perhaps think less about planning, frameworks, and intervention logics and more about how we create an environment that fosters compassion and develops confidence and self-esteem; more trust, less accountability for workers, fewer written words, and more emphasis on relationships and listening. If relationships are more important than specifications, an important question for service managers might be how can contracts be managed in a way that facilitates rather than hinders work at the coalface? And, for researchers, the questions that need exploring might be: at what point does loss of faith in the system result in people not participating in it; and what are the characteristics of effective health care workers, what support do they value most, and what environmental changes do they see as most helpful?

# About the contributors

**Michael Belgrave** is a Professor of History at Massey University's Albany campus. He is primarily interested in applied history through work with claimants before the Waitangi Tribunal, on health and social policy history and also on contemporary social service delivery.

**Win Bennett** is General Manager Planning, Funding and Performance at Hawkes Bay District Health Board. Interests are primary health care, managing complex change and interventions to reduce inequalities.

**Sarah Bierre** is a PhD student in the Department of Public Health at the University of Otago, Wellington. Her research interests include critical theories and methodologies, the determinants of inequalities in health and the relationships between housing policy, history, and public health.

**Julia Carr** is a public health physician and general practitioner whose main interest is primary health care. She is currently working in a planning and funding role within Capital & Coast DHB, Wellington.

**Peter Crampton** is Head of Department in the Department of Public Health at the University of Otago, Wellington. Peter is a specialist in public health medicine. His research is focused on social indicators and social epidemiology, health care policy, and primary health care organisation and funding.

**Chris Cunningham** is Professor of Māori Health at Massey University and Director of the Research Centre for Māori Health & Development. His research interests are in non-communicable disease, the longitudinal study of small collectives (whānau) and outcome measurement for ethnic groups.

**Kevin Dew** is an Associate Professor in the Department of Public Health, University of Otago, Wellington. He is a sociologist whose research interests include health inequalities, health communication and interaction.

**Brian Easton** is an independent scholar. His research interests include health systems, the evaluation of treatments and the social costs of illness, especially alcohol, tobacco and gambling. He has recently published *Globalisation and the Wealth of Nations*.

**Jon Foley** manages the System Performance team in the New Zealand Ministry of Health. From 2000 to 2005, he was involved in various aspects of the development and implementation of the Primary Health Care Strategy, including Primary Health Organisation (PHO) funding formulae, enrolment policy, performance management, and information systems.

**John Forman** is Executive Director of the New Zealand Organisation for Rare Disorders, a health and disability information and advocacy organisation. He has written and presented on family experience of rare genetic disease and on many aspects of health and disability policy, including ethics, medicine access, biotechnology, medical/social models, service provision and research.

**Maude Governor** is Māori Community Health Worker at Newtown Union Health Service in Wellington. She is passionate about reducing health inequalities by working towards enhancing the provision of health services through informing, connecting, engaging and responding to the health needs of Māori.

**Sarah Hill** is a public health physician and Senior Research Fellow in the Department of Public Health, University of Otago, Wellington. Her research interests include health inequalities, health services and social epidemiology.

**Philippa Howden-Chapman** is a social scientist and Professor in the Department of Public Health, University of Otago, Wellington. She is the Director of *He Kainga Oranga*/Housing and Health Research Programme, where she is principal investigator for the Housing, Insulation and Health Study, the Housing, Heating and Health Study, the Tokelau Extended Housing Study and the Housing (Dis)ability Study. She is a contributor to the WHO Housing Group in Bonn and the WHO Urban Settlements Group in Kobe.

**Kathy James** is a front line primary health care doctor working with high need populations in Aotearoa New Zealand. Her clinical interests are refugee health, mental health and developing improved services with and for Māori and Pacific communities locally. She is currently working for Newtown Union Health Service and in 2007 edited a book, *Health for the People – Newtown Union Health Service – 20 years on*.

**Olivia James** is a consultant, working mainly in South Auckland. Her interests include working with organisations to address health inequalities through community action.

**Anna Matheson** is a PhD student in the Department of Public Health, University of Otago, Wellington. Her research interests include community and policy interventions, health inequalities, complexity theory and methods, and the relationship between micro and macro social phenomena.

**Tim McCreanor** is a Pakeha member of Whariki Research Group, a Māori public health unit at Massey University in Auckland. His key interests are in research to support social change toward equity and social justice, focusing on discursive and qualitative research into race relations, identity and power.

**Lianne Ormsby** works at Maraeroa Marae Health Clinic in Waitangirua Porirua. She is a Tamariki Ora nurse and an Outreach Vaccinator and all her visits are in the home. After working in the hospital for sixteen years, she has found the community work much more rewarding as it gives her the opportunity to be involved with the whole whānau.

**Bridget Robson** (Ngati Raukawa) is Director of Te Rōpū Rangahau Hauora a Eru Pōmare (the Eru Pōmare Māori Health Research Centre) at the University of Otago, Wellington. Her research interests include the social determinants of health, disparities in access to and receipt of health care, and the development of kaupapa Māori epidemiology.

**Eugene Ryder** works for Wesley Community Action. His role is 'Rangatahi Support Worker' and he works under Mason Durie's 'Tapa-wha' model. Eugene has worked in the youth sector for over fifteen years. Mahi evolves around linking rangatahi and whānau to existing services. Target group is mainly, but not exclusive to, whānau who have been imprisoned, have links with gangs or gang members, have dropped out of school or have 'fallen through the system'. A key to Eugene's mahi is the fact that he comes from and belongs to the community that he is working with. With a wealth of experience, he is able to relate easily to the varying challenges that rangatahi and their whānau face.

**Susan St John** is a senior lecturer in economics and the co-director of the Retirement Policy and Research Centre, University of Auckland, researcher on family incomes in New Zealand, and executive member of the Child Poverty Action Group Inc.

**Louise Signal** is a Director of the Health Promotion and Policy Research Unit, University of Otago, Wellington. She is a social scientist whose research interests include addressing health inequalities, health promotion and the public health aspects of food.

**Maggie Simcox** is a practice nurse in Porirua. She has worked there for the last fifteen years, the last four of which she has specialised in Chronic Disease Management and she is passionate about this.

**Lee Tan** is a Senior Analyst with Capital & Coast DHB, whose interest is in managing data to provide meaningful information for health systems and communities.

# Notes

## Chapter 2

1 The mortality rates were age-standardised to the WHO population, while the CABG and angioplasty rates were age-standardised to the younger Segi's population. The point of this graph is to show the inverse patterns of mortality and heart procedure rates.

2 The list of amenable diseases included hypertensive heart disease; tuberculosis; asthma; chronic rheumatic heart disease; appendicitis; acute respiratory disease; bacterial infections; Hodgkin's disease; abdominal hernias; acute and chronic cholecystitis; deficiency anaemias; pneumonia and bronchitis (Sporle, Pearce & Davis 2002). Salmond & Crampton (2000) also report increasing gradients in potentially 'avoidable' mortality by area deprivation, with Māori rates higher than non-Māori at each deprivation decile among 25–44 and 45–64-year-old males and females – this classification includes a broader range of causes of death used by the Ministry of Health (1999).

3 Including GST, the tax take from Māori smokers would be $220m. Non-Māori smokers pay approximately $600m excise tax and $680m including GST.

4 Twenty-one per cent of Pākehā children live in restricted economic living standards compared to 49 per cent of Māori children and 42 per cent of Pacific children (Krishnan et al. 2002: 114). Thirteen per cent of Pākehā children (around 65,000) were in the lowest income quintile in 1996 compared to 34 per cent of Māori children (69,000) and 34 per cent of Pacific children (28,000) (CPAG 2003). Just under 19 per cent of 'economic families' with a European/Pākehā adult had net-of-housing-cost incomes below 60 per cent of median in 2000 compared to 32 per cent of families with a Māori adult and 40 per cent of families with a Pacific adult (Ministry of Social Development 2003) – note that the number of children within Māori and Pacific families will be higher on average than the number of children within Pākehā economic families. An economic family is 'a group of co-resident people whose financial affairs are common or have been merged to the extent the people are substantially interdependent' (Ministry of Social Development 2003: 147).

5 For example, among low-income families the average living standard scores are higher among Pākehā families than Māori families. Over two-

thirds (72 per cent) of Māori in 'sole-parent families' have scores in the ranges 'somewhat restricted' to 'very restricted', compared to 53 per cent of all people in sole-parent families (Krishnan *et al*. 2002).

6   Among European families, the proportion of families in the lowest income group decreases as the youngest child ages, but remains the same for Māori families (Horsfield & Evans 1988).

7   By the age of 14 years, Māori boys in the Christchurch Health and Development Study were twice as likely to come to police attention as non-Māori offenders with the same self-reported offending history and socio-economic status (Fergusson *et al*. 1993).

8   By the age of 21 years, Māori were 2.6 times more likely to be convicted of property offences, and 1.7 times more for all offences, than non-Māori with the same level of self-reported offending, educational status and socio-economic status (Fergusson *et al*. 2003a). For cannabis related offences, Māori with same level of cannabis use and history of contact with the police were four times more likely to be arrested than non-Māori with same characteristics, and four times more likely to be convicted. (Fergusson *et al*. 2003b)

# Chapter 3

1   Confusion often arises over the idea of a mortality rate or risk. 'Surely everyone dies eventually, so mortality must be 100 per cent in everyone!' An easy way of understanding mortality risk is to think of a person's risk of dying *in the next year*. If they belong to a population group with a mortality rate of 200 per 100,000 per year, their risk of dying in the next year is twice as high as that of someone whose population group has a mortality rate of 100 per 100,000 per year. Groups with higher mortality rates will have (correspondingly) lower life expectancy. In other words, higher mortality risk means a person is more likely to die earlier than someone in a lower risk group.

2   Previous research based on individual measures (such as that by Pearce and colleagues) relied heavily on occupational class as a marker of socio-economic position. Women are typically excluded from such analyses because a significant proportion are outside the paid workforce and cannot be assigned an occupational grouping – meaning studies are limited to men. Use of measures such as household income and educational status allows the study of socio-economic health inequalities to be extended to the other half of the population.

3   The Dunedin longitudinal study – or (to use its full name) the Dunedin Multidisciplinary Health and Development Study – is a study following a cohort of children from infancy into adulthood. The study includes all children born in the Dunedin area in a 12-month period during the early 1970s, and has followed their development over time into (currently) their early thirties (Silva & Stanton 1996).

4 'Household income' is a measure of the combined income of everyone living in the same household, usually adjusted ('equivalised') for the number of adults and children living in that household.

5 See Ministry of Health 2000, Appendix 3 for a more complete explanation of the Gini coefficient.

6 This can be tested by using a ruler or pen to make a line connecting the tops of the three columns in each group. As the ruler is moved across the graph it can be kept at the same angle and still connect the columns in each triplet.

7 Absolute inequality is the difference in height between the tallest and shortest columns.

8 Relative inequality is the height of the tallest column compared with (or divided by) the height of the shortest column.

9 For a more complete explanation of absolute and relative inequalities see Blakely et al. 2005.

10 If all households in New Zealand were placed along a continuum with lowest disposable income at one end and highest disposable income at the other, the household one-fifth of the way along this line would represent the 20th percentile (Household 20) and the household four fifths of the way along this line would represent the 80th percentile (Household 80). The *ratio of disposable household income* is then calculated by dividing disposable income in Household 80 by disposable income in Household 20. If disposable income was the same in both households, this ratio would be 1.0. The higher the ratio, the more unequal the distribution of disposable income.

# Chapter 4

1 *Te Hoe Nuku Roa* is funded by a grant from the Foundation for Research, Science & Technology.

2 Northland and Southland were added to the study in 2004/5 and feature only in the fourth longitudinal wave.

3 Outcomes were measured using a framework developed within the study – Te Ngahuru (Durie *et al.* 2003a) – which provides the context for specific outcomes and indicators in the fields of Māori and whānau wellbeing, culture and cultural identity, the Māori estate and Māori synergies.

4 *Oranga Kaumātua* is currently funded through a programme grant from the Health Research Council of New Zealand. The initial survey in 1997 was funded by Te Puni Kōkiri – Ministry of Māori Development and Massey University.

5 Respondents are initially recruited (non-randomly) through iwi networks, and following interviews are asked to suggest others who might also participate (sometimes called 'snowball' sampling).

6 The Māori world.

7 Oranga Kaumātua shows that fewer than half of older Māori have access to whānau; most live either alone or in a couple-only situation meaning

whānau-centric policies and practices are likely to exacerbate inequity if they are thought (naïvely) to be universally applicable.

8 See www.tuhono.net

9 Te Whare Tapa Wha likens hauora to a symmetrical, strong house, with four walls representing tinana (physical) wairua (spiritual) whānau (family) and hinengaro (mental) dimensions. Te Wheke likens hauora to an octopus with meanings ascribed to the body and tentacles and suckers. Ngā Pou Mana likens hauora to a carved pole (see Durie 1998).

# Chapter 6

1 I am indebted to Avril Bell (Bell 2004b) for this term, which I will use interchangeably with the more contested word Pākehā, which has nevertheless a strong popular usage meaning New Zealanders of European descent. I also use it to refer to what might elsewhere be known as 'mainstream' culture: the established, dominant institutions, practices and norms of society in this country.

# Chapter 8

1 The kind permission of David Fletcher to reproduce this cartoon is acknowledged.

2 It was even more ironic in that Ruth had already attacked the universal child benefit which was amalgamated with Family Support prior to the 1991 budget.

3 The figure for the lowest decile is an unreliable indicator of their access to resources. Expenditure in the lowest decile is much higher than declared income and may involve reported business losses, so that it is more usual to aggregate the bottom deciles.

4 Crude poverty line figures must be supplemented by other data, as they do not measure the extent of poverty or its duration for example. Surveys of living standards such as reported by the Ministry of Social Development and described in Perry (2004) can be useful in giving a fuller picture.

5 Estimates that take into account additional Working for Families spending for 2006 have not been made. This new spending does not affect the children in families on benefits.

6 This analysis focuses on children under 13 years of age. Older children have had a bigger increase in their Family Support, but have also suffered increases in user-pays costs for education.

7 See for example the Issues Paper for the 2001 Tax Review (McLeod 2001: 98).

8 For a full discussion of family tax credits in different countries see Nolan (Nolan 2004a).

9 There is a working tax credit in the UK but it is not confined to families, and most countries subsidise the costs of child care for those who are working.

10 Only about 6 per cent of children lose all the tax credits.

# Chapter 10

1 Deprived areas are determined using the New Zealand Deprivation Index (NZDep). The NZDep index of socio-economic deprivation is a census-based small-area index of deprivation (Salmond & Crampton 2002).

2 Typically, mortality rates are standardised by age, which is closely associated with mortality, to enable comparisons to be made between regions with different age profiles.

3 Nevertheless, changes in population had been used for many years, along with other factors, to determine resource allocation to hospital boards. In broad terms hospital boards had been funded according to the previous year's allocations, with adjustments for changes in population size, capital-driven commissioning grants, and increases in hospital bed days.

4 Health Care Aotearoa is a network of community-based, non-profit primary health care organisations that provide a range of health services primarily to Māori, Pacific, and residents of the most socio-economically deprived New Zealand communities.

5 'Cream skimming' is the practice of engaging in certain enrolment techniques to increase the likelihood of enrolling healthy people and, thereby, to reduce the risk that the health plan will incur expenditures above the prospective payment level.

6 Perverse incentives are unintended and counterproductive incentives, and moral hazard refers to provider (or patient) behaviour that is problematic or immoral because the provider (or patient) doesn't suffer the consequences of their behaviour.

7 The R squared value shows the portion of health care expenditure that is explained by the variables used in the risk rating formula; for example, an R squared of 0.183 means that 18.3 per cent of the variation is explained.

# Chapter 11

1 Ambulatory-sensitive hospitalisations are those which are sensitive to prophylactic or therapeutic interventions delivered in a primary health care setting, or through ambulatory services like outpatients, for example, early diagnosis, immunisation or screening.

2 The Primary Health Organisation system, initiated in the strategy and population-based payment system to support this, brought a new clarity about the population served by primary care providers, including each participating general practice. Demographic information for the enrolled population includes age, gender, ethnicity, NZDep (a small area measure of deprivation) and geocoding of address is also included. Before this, there was no system of enrolment and patients could be defined as part of the population served, or 'casual'( without any formality or consistency across providers).

3 Ministry of Health. *Healthy Eating – Healthy Action. Oranga Kai – Oranga Pumau. A strategic Framework.* Wellington: Ministry of Health 2003.

4   GMS refers to general medical and practice nurse subsidies which pre-
    dated the PHO capitation system of payment. GMS was an activity-based
    subsidy for eligible populations based on a per visit claim with a practice
    nurse subsidy based on a percentage of practice nurse hours. Capitation
    funding is funding paid regularly, according to a funding formula and
    dependent on a registered patient population.

## Chapter 12

1   *He Kainga Oranga* refers to 'some health housing', where *kainga* can
    mean both home and village, thus highlighting the broad scope of the
    Programme.

## Chapter 13

1   Discrimination against people with disabilities by the able-bodied.
2   Absolute inequalities are differences in mortality rates between low- and
    high-income people. Relative inequalities are the ratio of these mortality
    rates for low- compared to high-income people.
3   HIA is defined as 'a combination of procedures, methods and tools by
    which a policy, program or project may be assessed and judged for its
    potential effects on the health of the population, and the distribution of
    those effects within the population' (European Centre for Health Policy
    1999).
4   Although the Intervention Framework can be used independently of the
    HEAT tool, the HEAT tool incorporates the Intervention Framework and
    is therefore a compilation tool.

## Chapter 14

1   Alan Duff, *Once Were Warriors*. Auckland: Tandem Press, 1990; motion
    picture, 1994.
2   The Mantoux test is a test for TB infection. It involves injection of a protein
    extract (tuberculin) into the person's skin. A positive reaction – swelling
    of a designed size around the injection site after several days – indicates
    infection with TB at some time past or present. A negative reaction,
    however, does not necessarily mean the person does not have active TB
    disease.

## Chapter 15

1   The Health Inequalities and Need Symposium was held at Te Papa
    Tongarewa in Wellington on 27 August 2004.
2   In this context 'mainstream' refers to services that are delivered with the
    entire population in mind, but as such often deliver in ways that suit 'most'
    people. This can be a problem for particular groups of people and so as an
    alternative to mainstream services some services are 'targeted' or delivered
    with particular groups in mind.

# References

## Chapter 1

Bauld, L., Judge, K., Barnes, M., Benzeval, M., MacKenzie, M., Sullivan, H. (2005). 'Promoting social change: The experience of the Health Action Zones in England.' *Journal of Social Policy*, 34(3): 427–45.

Brunner, E., Marmot, M. (1999). 'Social organization, stress and health.' (ed. M. Marmot & R. Wilkinson). Oxford: Oxford University Press, pp. 17–43.

Craig, D., Porter, D. (2005). 'The third way and the third world: Poverty reduction and social inclusion strategies in the rise of "inclusive" liberalism.' *Review of International Political Economy*, 12(2): 226–63.

Evans, R. (2002). *Interpreting and Addressing Inequalities in Health: From Black to Acheson to Blair…?* London: Office of Health Economics.

Gray, D. (2006). *Health Sociology: An Australian Perspective*. French Forests (NSW): Pearson Education Australia.

Johansson, J. (2004). 'Orewa and the rhetoric of illusion.' *Political Science*, 56(2): 101–119.

Ministry of Health (2002). *Reducing Inequalities in Health*. Wellington: Ministry of Health.

Ministry of Social Policy (2001). *The Social Report 2001*. Wellington: Ministry of Social Policy.

O'Dea, D., Howden-Chapman, P. (2000). 'Income and income inequality and health.' In P. Howden-Chapman & M. Tobias (eds), *Social Inequalities in Health: New Zealand 1999*. Wellington: Ministry of Health, pp. 65–86.

Peters, M. (1997). 'Neoliberalism, welfare dependency and the moral construction of poverty in New Zealand.' *New Zealand Sociology*, 12(1): 1–34.

Roper, B.S. (2005). *Prosperity for All?: Economic, Social and Political Change in New Zealand since 1935*. Southbank, Vic: Thomson Learning.

Sorensen, G., Emmons, K., Hunt, M., Johnston, D. (1998). 'Implications of the results of community intervention trials.' *Annual Review of Public Health*, 19: 379–416.

World Health Organization (2006). *World Health Report 2006: Working Together for Health*. Geneva: World Health Organization.

## Chapter 2

Ajwani, S., Blakely, T., Robson, B., Tobias, M., Bonne, M. (2003). *Decades of Disparity: Ethnic Mortality Trends in New Zealand 1980–1999*. Wellington: Ministry of Health and University of Otago.

Alexander, W.R.J., Genc, M., Jaforullah, M. (2003). *Māori Disadvantage in the Labour Market*. Dunedin: Department of Economics, University of Otago.

Bhattacharyya, G., Gabriel, J., Small, S. (2002). *Race and Power: Global Racism in the Twenty-first Century*. London and New York: Routledge.

Carlson, D. (1997). 'Stories of colonial and postcolonial education.' In M. Fine, L. Weis, L. Powell, L.M. Wong (eds), *Off White: Readings on Race, Power, and Society*. New York, London: Routledge, pp. 135–46.

Child Poverty Action Group Inc. (2003). *Our Children: The Priority for Policy*. (2nd edn). Auckland: Child Poverty Action Group Inc.

Crampton, P., Salmond, C., Woodward, A., Reid, P. (2000). 'Socioeconomic deprivation and ethnicity are both important for anti-tobacco health promotion.' *Health Education & Behavior*, 27: 317–27.

Cunningham, C., Durie, M., Fergusson, D., Fitzgerald, E., Hong, B., Horwood, J., Jensen, J., Rochford, M., Stevenson, B. (2002). *Ngā Āhuatanga Noho o te Hunga Pakeke Māori: Living Standards of Older Māori 2002*. Wellington. Ministry of Social Development.

Davis P., McLeod K., Ransom M., Ongley P. (1997). The New Zealand Socioeconomic Index of Occupational Status (NZSEI). Research Report No 2. Wellington: Statistics New Zealand.

Dovidio, J. (1997). 'Aversive racism and the need for affirmative action.' Reprinted in K. Reilly, S. Kaufama, A. Bodino (eds), *Racism: A Global Reader*. New York: M.E. Sharpe.

D'Souza, A., Wood, E. (2003). 'Healthy Lives.' *Making New Zealand Fit for Children: Promoting a National Plan of Action for New Zealand Children*. Wellington: UNICEF New Zealand.

Fergusson, D., Horwood, L., Ynskey, M. (1993). 'Ethnicity, social background and young offending: A 14 year longitudinal study.' *Australian and New Zealand Journal of Criminology*, 26: 155–170.

Fergusson, D., Swain-Campbell, N., Horwood, J. (2003a). *Is There Ethnic Bias in Conviction Rates in New Zealand?* Christchurch: Christchurch Health and Development Study, Christchurch School of Medicine.

Fergusson, D., Swain-Campbell, N., Horwood, J. (2003b). *Arrests and Convictions for Cannabis Related Offences in a New Zealand Birth Cohort*. Christchurch: Christchurch Health and Development Study, Christchurch School of Medicine.

Gaertner, S., Dovidio, J., Banker, B. (1997). 'Does white racism necessarily mean antiblackness? Aversive racism and prowhiteness.' In M. Fine, L. Weis, L. Powell, L.M. Wong (eds), *Off White: Readings on Race, Power, and Society*. New York, London: Routledge, pp. 167–78.

Horsfield, A., Evans, M. (1988). *Māori Women in the Economy: A Preliminary Review of the Economic Position of Māori Women in New Zealand*. Wellington: Te Ohu Whakatupu, Te Minitatanga mō ngā Wāhine.

Howden-Chapman, P., Wilson, N. (2000). 'Housing and health.' In P. Howden-Chapman, M. Tobias (eds), *Social Inequalities in Health: New Zealand 1999*. Wellington: Ministry of Health, pp. 133–45.

Howell, G., Hackwell, K. (2003). *Why don't Māori and Pacific Children get the Disability Allowance?* Wellington: Downtown Community Ministry.

Jarvis, M., Wardle, J. (1999). 'Social patterning of individual health behaviours: The case of cigarette smoking.' In M. Marmot, R. Wilkinson (eds), *Social Determinants of Health*. Oxford: Oxford University Press, pp. 240–55.

Jeffries, R. (1998). *Māori Participation in Tertiary Education. Barriers and Strategies to Overcome Them.* Wellington: Te Puni Kōkiri.

Krishnan, V., Jensen, J., Ballantyne, S. (2002). *New Zealand Living Standards 2000: Ngā Āhuatanga Noho o Aotearoa.* Wellington: Ministry of Social Development.

Laugesen, M., Clements, M. (1998). *Cigarette Smoking Mortality among Māori, 1954–2028.* Wellington: Te Puni Kōkiri.

Macdonald, J. (1986). *Racism and Rental Accommodation: A Report of the Office of the Race Relations Conciliator.* Auckland: Race Relations Office.

Māori Women's Housing Research Project (1991). '... *for the sake of decent shelter* ...' Wellington: Housing Corporation of New Zealand.

McCracken, S., Feyer, A., Langley, J., Broughton, J., Sporle, A. (2001). 'Māori work-related fatal injury, 1985–1994.' *New Zealand Medical Journal*, 114: 395–9.

McCreanor, T., Nairn, R. (2002). 'Tauiwi general practitioners talk about Māori health interpretative repertoires.' *New Zealand Medical Journal*, 115: 1–8.

Ministry of Health (1999). *Our Health, Our Future. Hauora Pakari, Koiora Roa: The Health of New Zealanders 1999.* Wellington: Ministry of Health.

Ministry of Health (2001). *Inhaling Inequality: Tobacco's Contribution to Health Inequality in New Zealand.* Wellington: Ministry of Health.

Ministry of Social Development (2003). *The Social Report 2003.* Wellington: Ministry of Social Development.

Minitatanga mō ngā Wāhine (2002). *Mahi Orite, Utu Tokeke. Pay Equity for Women.* Wellington: Minitatanga mō ngā Wāhine.

National Research Bureau (1996). *Environmental Tobacco Smoke Study 1996: A Report for the Ministry of Health.* Wellington: National Research Bureau Ltd.

New Zealand Health Information Service (2004). *Suicide Facts. Provisional 2001 Statistics (all ages).* Wellington: New Zealand Health Information Service.

Nolte, E., McKee, M. (2003). 'Measuring the health of nations: Analysis of mortality amenable to health care.' *British Medical Journal*, 327: 1129.

O'Dea, D., Howden-Chapman, P. (2000). 'Income and income inequality and health'. In P. Howden-Chapman, M. Tobias (eds), *Social Inequalities in Health: New Zealand 1999*. Wellington: Ministry of Health, pp. 65–86.

Pearce, N.E., Davis, P.B., Smith, A.H., Foster, F.H. (1984). 'Mortality and social class in New Zealand III: Male mortality by ethnic group', *New Zealand Medical Journal*, 97: 31–5.

Pearce, N., Pōmare, E., Marshall, S., Borman, B. (1993). 'Mortality and social class in Māori and non-Māori New Zealand men: Changes between 1975–77 and 1985–87.' *New Zealand Medical Journal*, 106: 193–6.

Pōmare, E., Keefe-Ormsby, V., Ormsby, C., Pearce, N., Reid, P., Robson, B., Wātene-Haydon, N. (1995). *Hauora: Māori Standards of Health. A Study of the Years 1970–1991.* Wellington: Te Rōpū Rangahau Hauora a Eru Pōmare.

Pool, I. (1991). *Te Iwi Māori: A New Zealand Population Past, Recent and Projected.* Auckland: Auckland University Press.

Reid, P., Pouwhare, R. (1991). *Te Taonga-mai-Tawhiti: The Gift from a Distant Place.* Auckland: Niho Taniwha.

Salmond, C., Crampton, P. (2000). 'Deprivation and health.' In P. Howden-Chapman, M. Tobias (eds), *Social Inequalities in Health: New Zealand 1999.* Wellington: Ministry of Health, pp. 9–63.

Shaw, M., Dorling, D., Gordon, D., Davey Smith, G. (1999). *The Widening Gap: Health Inequalities and Policy in Britain.* Bristol: The Policy Press.

Smith, A.H., Pearce, N.E. (1984). 'Determinants of differences in mortality between New Zealand Māori and non-Māori aged 15–64.' *New Zealand Medical Journal*, 197: 101–8.

Sporle, A., Pearce, N., Davis, P. (2002). 'Social class differences in Māori and non-Māori aged 15–64 during the last two decades.' *New Zealand Medical Journal*, 115: 127–31.

Sutherland, H., Alexander, R. (2002). *The Occupational Distribution of Māori 1997–2000.* Dunedin: Department of Economics, University of Otago.

Te Puni Kōkiri (2000). *Māori in the New Zealand Economy.* (2nd edn). Wellington: Te Puni Kōkiri.

Te Puni Kōkiri (2001). *The Quality of Teacher Training for Teaching Māori Students.* Wellington: Te Puni Kōkiri.

Tipene-Leach, D., Abel, S., Finau, S., Park, J., Lenna, M. (2000). 'Māori infant care practices: Implications for health messages, infant care services and SIDS prevention in Māori communities.' *Pacific Health Dialog*, 7: 29–37.

Tukuitonga, C., Bindman, A. (2002). 'Ethnic and gender differences in the use of coronary artery revascularisation procedures in New Zealand.' *New Zealand Medical Journal*, 115: 179–82.

van Ryn, M., Burke, J. (2000). 'The effect of patient race and socio-economic status on physicians' perceptions of patients.' *Social Science and Medicine*, 50: 813–28.

Westbrooke, I., Baxter, J., Hogan, J. (2000). 'Are Māori under-served for cardiac interventions?' *New Zealand Medical Journal*, 114: 484–7.

Wilson, N. (2000a). 'Occupational Class and Health.' In P. Howden-Chapman, M. Tobias (eds), *Social Inequalities in Health: New Zealand 1999.* Wellington: Ministry of Health, pp. 103–18.

Wilson, N. (2000b). 'Labour Force Status and Health.' In P. Howden-Chapman, M. Tobias (eds), *Social Inequalities in Health: New Zealand 1999.* Wellington: Ministry of Health, pp. 119–32.

# Chapter 3

Ajwani, S., Blakely, T., Robson, B., Tobias, M., Bonne, M. (2003). *Decades of Disparity: Ethnic Mortality Trends in New Zealand 1980–1999*. Wellington: Ministry of Health. http://www.wnmeds.ac.nz/nzcms-info.html

Barnett, R., Pearce, J., Moon, G. (2005). 'Does social inequality matter? Changing ethnic socio-economic disparities and Māori smoking in New Zealand, 1981–1996.' *Social Science & Medicine*, 60: 1515–26.

Berkman, L.S., Kawachi, I. (eds), (2000). *Social Epidemiology*. New York: Oxford University Press.

Black D., Morris J., Smith C., Townsend P. (1980). *Inequalities in Health: Report of a Research Working Group*. London: Department of Health & Social Security.

Borman, B., de Boer, G., Fraser, J. (1990). 'Risk factors for low birthweight in New Zealand, 1981–83.' *New Zealand Medical Journal*, 103: 92–4.

Borman, B., Wilson, N., Mailing, C. (1999). 'Socio-demographic characteristics of New Zealand smokers: Results from the 1996 census.' *New Zealand Medical Journal*, 112: 460–3.

Blakely, T. (2002a). *The New Zealand Census – Mortality Study: Socio-economic Inequalities and Adult Mortality 1991–94*. Wellington: Ministry of Health.

Blakely, T., Kiro, C., Woodward, A. (2002b). 'Unlocking the numerator-denominator bias II: Adjustments to mortality rates by ethnicity and deprivation during 1991–94.' *New Zealand Medical Journal*, 115: 43–8.

Blakely, T., Fawcett, J., Atkinson, J., Tobias, M., Cheung, J. (2005). *Decades of Disparity II: Socio-economic Mortality Trends in New Zealand, 1981–1999*. Wellington: Ministry of Health.

Collins, D.C.A., Kearns, R. (2005). 'Geographies of inequality: Child pedestrian injury and walking school buses in Auckland, New Zealand.' *Social Science & Medicine*, 60: 61–9.

Copplestone, J.F., Rose, R.J. (1967). *Occupational Mortality Among Male Population, Other than Māori, 20 to 64 Years of Age*. Wellington: Department of Health.

Crampton, P., Salmond, C., Sutton, F. (1997a). 'NZDep91: A new index of deprivation.' *Social Policy Journal of New Zealand*, 9: 186–93.

Crampton, P., Howden-Chapman, P. (1997b). *Socio-economic Inequalities and Health. Proceedings of the Socio-economic Inequalities & Health Conference, 9–10 December 1996, Wellington*. Institute of Policy Studies, Wellington, New Zealand.

Crampton, P., Salmond, C., Woodward, A., Reid, P. (2000). 'Socio-economic deprivation and ethnicity are both important for anti-tobacco health promotion.' *Health Education & Behaviour*, 3: 317–27.

Davey Smith, G., Blane, D., Bartley, M. (1994). 'Explanations for socio-economic differences in mortality: Evidence from Britain and elsewhere.' *European Journal of Public Health*, 4(2): 131–44.

Davey Smith, G., Shaw, M., Dorling D., Pearce, N. (2002). 'The international evidence.' In Pearce N., Ellison-Loschmann, L. (eds), *Explanations for Socio-economic Differences in Health: Proceedings from the First Annual CPHR Symposium in Health Research & Policy*. Wellington: Centre for Public Health Research, Massey University (Wellington Campus), pp. 9–28.

Davis P., Graham P., Pearce, N. (1999). 'Health expectancy in New Zealand, 1981–1991: social variations and trends in a period of rapid social and economic change.' *Journal of Epidemiology & Community Health*, 53: 519–27.

Dharmalingam, A., Pool, I., Baxendine, S., Sceats, J. (2004). 'Trends and patterns of avoidable hospitalisations in New Zealand: 1980–1997.' *New Zealand Medical Journal*, 117: 1198. http://www.nzma.org.nz/journal/117-1198/976/

Elley, W.B., Irving, J.C. (1972). 'A socio-economic index for New Zealand based on levels of education and income from the 1996 census.' *New Zealand Journal of Educational Studies*, 2(2): 153–7.

Elley, W.B., Irving, J.C. (1976). 'Revised socio-economic index for New Zealand.' *New Zealand Journal of Educational Studies*, 11(1): 25-36.

Fawcett, J., Blakely, T., Robson, B., Tobias, M., Harris, R., PakiPaki, N. (2006). *Decades of Disparity III: Ethnic and Socio-economic Inequalities in Mortality, New Zealand 1981–1999*. Wellington: Ministry of Health.

Harris, R., Tobias, M., Jeffreys, M., Waldegrave, K., Karson, S., Nazroo, J. (2006). 'Effects of self-reported racial discrimination and deprivation on Māori health and inequalities in New Zealand: Cross-sectional study.' *The Lancet*, 367: 2005–2009.

Hefford, M., Crampton, P., Foley, J. (2005). 'Reducing health disparities through primary care reform: The New Zealand experiment.' *Health Policy*, 72: 9–23.

Hill, S.E., Blakely, T., Howden-Chapman, P. (2003). *Smoking Inequalities: Policies and Patterns of Inequality in New Zealand, 1981–96*. Wellington: Ministry of Health.

Howden-Chapman, P., Tobias, M. (eds) (2000). *Social Inequalities in Health: New Zealand 1999*. Wellington: Ministry of Health.

Jackson, G., Tobias, M. (2001). 'Potentially avoidable hospitalisations in New Zealand, 1989–98.' *Australian & New Zealand Journal of Public Health*, 25(3): 212–21.

Kawachi, I., Marshall, S., Pearce, N. (1991). 'Social class inequalities in the decline of coronary health disease among New Zealand men, 1975–77 and 1985–87.' *International Journal of Epidemiology*, 20(2): 393–8.

King, A. (2000). *The New Zealand Health Strategy*. Wellington: Ministry of Health.

King, A. (2001). *The Primary Health Care Strategy*. Wellington: Ministry of Health.

Lopez, A.D., Collishaw, N.E., Piha, T. (1994). 'A descriptive model of the cigarette epidemic in developed countries.' *Tobacco Control*, 3: 242–7.

Macintyre, S. (1997). 'The Black Report and beyond: What are the issues?' *Social Science & Medicine*, 44: 723–45.

Mackenbach, J., Bakker, M. (eds) (2002). *Reducing Inequalities in Health: A European Perspective*. London: Routledge.

Marmot, M. (1999). 'Introduction.' In Marmot, M. and Wilkinson, R.G. (eds), *Social Determinants of Health*. Oxford: Oxford University Press, pp. 1–16.

Marmot, M.G., Rose, G., Shipley, M., Hamilton, P.J. (1978). 'Employment grade and coronary heart disease in British civil servants.' *Journal of Epidemiology & Community Health*, 32: 244–49.

Marshall, S.W., Kawachi, I., Pearce, N., Borman, B. (1993). 'Social class differences in mortality from diseases amenable to medical intervention in New Zealand.' *International Journal of Epidemiology*, 22(2): 255–61.

McFadden, K., McConnell, D., Salmond, C., Crampton, P., Fraser, J. (2004). 'Socio-economic deprivation and the incidence of cervical cancer in New Zealand: 1988–1998.' *New Zealand Medical Journal*, 117: 1206. http://www.nzma.org.nz/journal/117-1206/1172/

Ministry of Health (2000). *Social Inequalities in Health: New Zealand 1999*. Wellington: Ministry of Health.

Ministry of Health (2002). *Reducing Inequalities in Health*. Wellington: Ministry of Health.

Ministry of Health (2004a). *A Portrait of Health: Key Results of the 2002/03 New Zealand Health Survey*. Wellington: Ministry of Health.

Ministry of Health (2004b). Chapter 9, 'Effectiveness.' In *The Health and Independence Report 2004: Director-General of Health's Annual Report on the State of Public Health 2005*. Wellington: Ministry of Health.

Ministry of Health (2005). Section 3.4, 'Effectiveness.' In *The Annual Report for the Year 2004/05 including The Health and Independence Report: Director-General of Health's Annual Report on the State of Public Health*. Wellington: Ministry of Health.

Ministry of Social Development (2005). *The Social Report 2005*. Wellington: Ministry of Social Development.

National Health Committee (1998). *The Social, Cultural and Economic Determinants of Health in New Zealand: Action to Improve Health*. Wellington: National Advisory Committee on Health & Disability.

O'Dea, D., Howden-Chapman, P. (2000). 'Income and income inequality and health.' In Howden-Chapman P., Tobias M. (eds), *Social Inequalities in Health: New Zealand 1999*. Wellington: Ministry of Health, pp. 65–86.

Pamuk, E., Makuc, D., Heck, K., Reuben, C., Lochner, K. (1998). *Socio-economic Status and Health Chartbook. Health, United States, 1998*. Maryland, USA: National Centre for Health Statistics.

Pearce, N., Davis, P.B., Smith, A.H., Foster, F.H. (1983a). 'Mortality and social class in New Zealand I: Overall male mortality.' *New Zealand Medical Journal*, 96(730): 281–5.

Pearce, N., Davis, P.B., Smith, A.H., Foster, F.H. (1983b). 'Mortality and social class in New Zealand II: Male mortality by major disease groupings.' *New Zealand Medical Journal*, 96(730): 281–5.

Pearce, N.E., Howard, J.K. (1986). 'Occupation, social class and male cancer mortality in New Zealand, 1974–78.' *International Journal of Epidemiology*, 15(4): 456–62.

Pearce, N., Marshall, S., Borman, B. (1991). 'Undiminished social class mortality differences in New Zealand men.' *New Zealand Medical Journal*, 104: 153–6.

Pearce, N., Pomare, E., Marshall, S., Borman, B. (1993). 'Mortality and social class in Māori and non-Māori New Zealand men: Changes between 1975–7 and 1985–7.' *New Zealand Medical Journal*, 106: 193–6.

Pearce, N., Bethwaite, P. (1997). 'Social class male cancer mortality in New Zealand, 1984–7.' *New Zealand Medical Journal*, 110(1045): 200–2.

Pearce, N., Ellison-Loschmann, L. (eds) (2002). *Explanations for Socio-economic Differences in Health: Proceedings from the First Annual CPHR Symposium in Health Research & Policy*. Wellington: Centre for Public Health Research, Massey University (Wellington Campus).

Pearce, N., Davis, P., Sporle, A. (2002). 'Persistent social class mortality differences in New Zealand men aged 15–64: An analysis of mortality during 1995–97.' *Australian & New Zealand Journal of Public Health*, 26: 17–22.

Poulton, R., Caspi, A., Milne, B.J., Thomson, W.M., Taylor, A., Sears, M.R., Moffit, T.E. (2002). 'Association between children's experience of socio-economic disadvantage and adult health: A life-course study.' *The Lancet*, 360(9346): 1640–5.

Reid, P., Robson, B., Jones, C.P. (2000). 'Disparities in health: Common myths and uncommon truths.' *Pacific Health Dialog*, 7(1): 38–47.

Riddell, T. (2005). 'Heart failure hospitalisations and deaths in New Zealand: Patterns by deprivation and ethnicity.' *New Zealand Medical Journal*, 118: 1208. http://www.nzma.org.nz/journal/117-1208/1254/

Roberts, I., Norton, R., Tuau, B. (1996). 'Child pedestrian injury rates: The importance of "exposure to risk" relating to socio-economic and ethnic differences, in Auckland, New Zealand.' *Journal of Epidemiology & Community Health*, 50: 162–5.

Robson, B. (2004). *Economic Determinants of Māori Health and Disparities*. Te Rōpū Rangahau Hauora a Eru Pōmare. Wellington: Wellington School of Medicine & Health Sciences, University of Otago.

Rose, G., Marmot, M.G. (1981). 'Social class and coronary heart disease.' *British Heart Journal*, 45: 13–19.

Salmond, C., Crampton, P., Sutton, F. (1998). 'NZDep91: A New Zealand index of deprivation.' *Australian & New Zealand Journal of Public Health*, 22(7): 835–7.

Salmond, C., Crampton, P., Hales, S., Lewis, S., Pearce, N. (1999). 'Asthma prevalence and deprivation: A small area analysis.' *Journal of Epidemiology & Community Health*, 53(8): 476–80.

Salmond, C., Crampton, P. (2000). 'Deprivation and health.' In Howden-Chapman, P., Tobias, M. (eds), *Social Inequalities in Health: New Zealand 1999*. Wellington: Ministry of Health, pp. 9-63.

Shaw, C., Blakely, T., Atkinson, J., Crampton, P. (2005a). 'Do social and economic reforms change socio-economic inequalities in child mortality? A case study: New Zealand 1981–1999.' *Journal of Epidemiology & Community Health*, 59(8): 638–44.

Shaw, C., Blakely, T., Sarfati, C., Fawcett, J., Hill, S. (2005b). 'Varying evolution of the New Zealand lung cancer epidemic by ethnicity and socio-economic position (1981–1999).' *New Zealand Medical Journal*, 118: 1213. http://www.nzma.org.nz/journal/118-1213/1411/

Shaw, C., Blakely, T., Crampton, P., Atkinson, J. (2005c). 'The contribution of causes of death to socio-economic inequalities in child mortality: New Zealand 1981–1999.' *New Zealand Medical Journal*, 118: 1227. http://www.nzma.org.nz/journal/118-1227/1779/

Shaw C., Blakely T., Sarfati D., Fawcett J., Pearce, J. (2006). 'Trends in colorectal cancer mortality by ethnicity and socio-economic position in New Zealand, 1981–99: One country, many stories.' *Australian & New Zealand Journal of Public Health*, 30(1): 64–70.

Silva, P.A., Stanton, W.R. (eds) (1996). *From Child to Adult: The Dunedin Multidisciplinary Health and Development Study*. Oxford: Oxford University Press.

Sporle, A., Pearce, N., Davis, P. (2002). 'Social class mortality differences in Māori and non-Māori men aged 15–64 during the last two decades.' *New Zealand Medical Journal*, 115: 127–31.

Taylor, W., Smeets, L., Hall, J., McPherson, K. (2004). 'The burden of rheumatic disorders in general practice: Consultation rates for rheumatic disease and the relationship to age, ethnicity, and small-area deprivation.' *New Zealand Medical Journal*, 117: 1203. http://www.nzma.org.nz/journal/118-1203/1298/

Victora, C.G., Vaughan, J.P., Barros, F.C., Silva, A.C., Tomasi, E. (2000). 'Explaining trends in inequities: Evidence from Brazilian child health studies.' *The Lancet*, 356: 1093–8.

Whitlock, G., MacMahon, S., Vander Hoorn, S., Davis, P., Jackson, R., Norton, R. (1997). 'Socio-economic distribution of smoking in a population of 10,529 New Zealanders.' *New Zealand Medical Journal*, 110: 327–30.

Whitlock, G., Norton, R., Clark, T., Pledger, M., Jackson, R., MacMahon, S. (2003). 'Motor vehicle driver injury and socio-economic status: A cohort study with prospective and retrospective driver injuries.' *Journal of Epidemiology & Community Health*, 57(7): 512–6.

Wilkinson, R.G. (1996). *Unhealthy Societies. The Afflictions of Inequality*. London: Routledge.

Wilkinson, R.G. (1999). 'Putting the picture together: Prosperity, redistribution, health and welfare.' In Marmot, M., Wilkinson, R.G. (eds), *Social Determinants of Health*. Oxford: Oxford University Press, pp. 256–74.

Williams, D.R. (1997). 'Race and health: basic questions, emerging directions.' *Annals of Epidemiology*, 7: 322–333.

## Chapter 4

Ajwani, S., Blakely, T., Robson, B., Tobias, M., & Bonne, M. (2003). *Decades of Disparity: Ethnic Mortality Trends in New Zealand 1980–1999*. Wellington: Ministry of Health.

Cunningham, C.W. (2004). 'The New Māori and Māori Health (Inaugural Professorial Lecture and 2004 Whanganui-a-Tara Lecture for Te Mata o Te Tau).' Wellington: Research Centre for Māori Health & Development, Massey University.

Cunningham, C.W., Fitzgerald, E., Stevenson, B. (2005). 'Pathways to Employment: An Analysis of Young Māori Workers *(Research Report 3/2005)*.' Wellington: Labour Market Dynamics Research Programme, Massey University.

Duric, M.H. (1994a). 'Kaupapa Hauora Māori: Policies for Māori Health.' (Paper presented at the Hui Te Ara Ahu Whakamua: Māori Health Decade Conference, Te Papaiouru Marae, Rotorua.

Durie, M.H. (1994b). 'Whanau, Whanaungatanga and Healthy Development.' (Paper presented at the Public Health Association Conference 1 June 1994, Palmerston North), Palmerston North: Department of Maori Studies, Massey University.

Durie, M.H. (1995). 'Nga Matatini Māori: Diverse Māori Realities.' (A Paper Prepared for the Ministry of Health). Palmerston North: Department of Māori Studies, Massey University.

Durie, M.H. (1998). *Whaiora: Māori Health Development* (2nd edn). Auckland: Oxford University Press.

Durie, M.H., Fitzgerald, E., Kingi, T.K.R., McKinley, S., Stevenson, B. (2002). *Māori Specific Outcomes and Indicators*. Palmerston North: School of Māori Studies, Massey University.

Durie, M., Fitzgerald, E., Kingi, T. K., McKinley, S., Brendan, S. (2003a). *Te Ngahura: A Māori Outcome Framework*. Palmerston North: School of Māori Studies, Massey University.

Durie, M.H., Fitzgerald, E.D.H., Stevenson, B., Kingi, T.K.R., McKinley, S. (2003b). 'Māori Outcome Indicators (A Report for the Ministry of Māori Development).' Wellington: Massey University.

Health Research Council of New Zealand (1998). *Rangahau Hauora Māori – Māori Health Research Themes 1998*. Auckland: HRC.

Metge, J. (1995). *New Growth from Old*. Wellington: Victoria University Press.

Ministry of Social Development (2004). 'New Zealand families today (A briefing for the Families Commission)'. Wellington: Ministry of Social Development.

Moeke-Pickering, T. (1996). Māori Identity: Whānau Identity. Unpublished Master of Social Science, University of Waikato.

Pōmare, E., Keefe-Ormsby, V., Ormsby, C., Pearce, N., Reid, P., Robson, B., Wātene-Haydon, N. (1995). *Hauora Maori Standards of Health III – A Study of the Years 1970–1991.* Wellington: Te Rōpu Rangahau Hauora a Eru Pomare, Wellington School of Medicine.

Smith, G. (1995). 'Whakaoho Whānau Ohanga: The Economics of Whānau as an Innovative Intervention into Māori Cultural and Educational Crises.' *He Pukenga Kōrero*, 1(1), 18.

Statistics New Zealand (2005). 'Understanding and Working with Ethnicity Data (Technical Paper).' Wellington: Statistics New Zealand.

Te Hoe Nuku Roa Research Team (1999). 'Te Hoe Nuku Roa Source Document: Baseline History.' Palmerston North: School of Māori Studies, Massey University.

## Chapter 5

Belgrave, M. (1991). 'Medicine and the rise of the health professions.' In L. Bryder (ed.), *A Healthy Country: Essays on the Social History of Medicine in New Zealand.* Wellington: Bridget Williams Books.

Belgrave, M. (2000). *The Mater: A History of Auckland's Mercy Hospital 1900–2000.* Palmerston North: Dunmore Press.

Belgrave, M. (2004). 'Needs and the state: Evolving social policy in New Zealand.' In B. Dalley and M. Tennant (eds), *Past Judgement: Social Policy in New Zealand History.* Dunedin: University of Otago Press.

Blair, T. (1998). *The Third Way: New Politics for the New Century.* London: Fabian Society.

Brunton, W.A. (2001). A choice of difficulties: National mental health policy in New Zealand, 1840–1947. Ph.D. thesis, University of Otago.

Bryder, L. (2003). *A Voice for Mothers: The Plunket Society and Infant Welfare, 1907–2000.* Auckland: Auckland University Press.

Cheyne, C., O'Brien, M., and Belgrave, M. (2004). *Social Policy in Aotearoa/ New Zealand: A Critical Introduction.* Auckland: Oxford University Press.

Dow, D.A. (1995). *Safeguarding the Public Health: A History of the New Zealand Department of Health.* Wellington: Victoria University Press in association with the Ministry of Health and with the assistance of the Historical Branch Dept. of Internal Affairs.

Easton, B. (1997). *The Commercialisation of New Zealand.* Auckland: Auckland University Press.

Easton, B. (1997a). *In Stormy Seas: The Post-War New Zealand Economy.* Dunedin: University of Otago Press.

Esping-Anderson, G. (1991). *The Three Worlds of Welfare Capitalism.* Cambridge: Polity Press.

Fairburn, M., and Olssen, E. (2005). *Class, Gender and the Vote: Historical Perspectives from New Zealand.* Dunedin: Otago University Press.

Fougere, G., Sharp, A., and University of Auckland (1992). *The Role of the State in the Health of the Nation.* Auckland: University of Auckland.

Giddens, A. (2000). *The Third Way: The Renewal of Social Democracy.* Malden, Mass.: Polity Press.

Hanson, E. (1980). *The Politics of Social Security. The 1938 Act and Some Later Developments.* Auckland: Auckland University Press/Oxford University Press.

Jamieson, J.P.S. (1941). *The Medical Profession and Social Security Medical Services.* Wellington: Commercial Printing and Pub. Co.

Kiro, C.A. (2001). Māori health policy and practice: Kimihia hauora Māori: Ngapuhi, Ngati-Hine, Ngati Te Rangiwewehe. Ph.D. Thesis, Massey University.

Mein Smith, P. (1986). *Maternity in Dispute: New Zealand, 1920–1939.* Wellington: Historical Publications Branch Dept. of Internal Affairs.

Oliver, W.H. (1977). 'The Origins and Growth of the Welfare State' in A.D. Trlin (ed.), *Social Welfare and New Zealand Society.* Wellington: Methuen New Zealand.

Oliver, W.II. (1979). 'Social Policy in the Liberal Period.' *New Zealand Journal of History* 13(1): 25–32.

Powell, M.A. (1999). *New Labour, New Welfare State?: The 'Third Way' in British Social Policy.* Bristol: Policy.

Rice, G. (1988). 'The making of New Zealand's 1920 Health Act.' *New Zealand Journal of History*, 22(1): 3–22.

Rice, G., Bryder, L. (2005). *Black November: The 1918 Influenza Pandemic in New Zealand.* Christchurch: Canterbury University Press.

Roper, B.S. (2005). *Prosperity for All?: Economic, Social and Political Change in New Zealand Since 1935.* Southbank, Vic.: Thomson Learning.

Shorter, E. (1991). *Doctors and their Patients: A Social History.* New Brunswick: Transaction Publishers.

Smith, F.B. (1988). *The Retreat of Tuberculosis, 1850–1950.* London and New York: Croom Helm.

Smith, F.B. (1993). *The People's Health, 1830–1910.* Aldershot, Hampshire: Gregg Revivals.

Smith, P.A. (2000). *The Private Prescription: The story of Southern Cross Health Care.* Auckland: Southern Cross Health Care.

Steel, F. (2005). 'A source of our wealth, yet adverse to our health? Butter and the diet-heart link in New Zealand to c.1990.' *Social History of Medicine*, 18(2): 475–93.

Tennant, M. (1979).'Duncan MacGregor and charitable aid administration 1886–1896.' *New Zealand Journal of History*, 13(1): 33–42.

Tennant, M. (1994). *Children's Health, the Nation's Wealth: A History of Children's Health Camps.* Wellington: Bridget Williams Books and Historical Branch, Dept. of Internal Affairs.

# Chapter 6

Abel, S. (1997). *Shaping the News: Waitangi Day on Television.* Auckland: Auckland University Press.

Adams, P. (1977). *Fatal Necessity: British Intervention in New Zealand 1830–1847*. Oxford: Oxford University Press.

Ajwani, S., Blakely, T., Robson, B., Tobias, M., Bonne, M. (2003). *Decades of Disparity: Ethnic Mortality Trends in New Zealand 1980–1999*. Wellington: Ministry of Health and University of Otago.

Anderson, B. (1991). *Imagined Communities* (rev. edn). London: Verso.

Antonovsky, A. (1996). 'The salutogenic model as a theory to guide health promotion'. *Health Promotion International*, 11: 11–18.

Armstead, C., Lawler, K., Gordon, G., Cross, J., Gibbons, J. (1989). 'Relationship of racial stressors to blood pressure and anger expression in black college students.' *Health Psychology*, 8: 541–56.

Ballara, A. (1986). *Proud To Be White: A Survey of Racial Prejudice in New Zealand*. Auckland: Heinemann.

Banks, J. (1962). *The Endeavour Journal of Joseph Banks 1768–1771*. Sydney: Trustees of the Public Library of New South Wales.

Beaglehole, J. (1968). *The Journals of Captain James Cook. VI*. Cambridge: Cambridge University Press.

Belich, J. (1986). *The New Zealand Wars and the Victorian Interpretation of Racial Conflict*. Auckland: Auckland University Press.

Belich, J. (1996). *Making Peoples: A History of the New Zealanders from Polynesian Settlement to the End of the Nineteenth Century*. Auckland: Penguin.

Bell, A. (1996). '"We're just New Zealanders": Pakeha identity politics.' In P. Spoonley, C. Macpherson, and D. Pearson (eds), *Nga Patai: Racism and Ethnic Relations in Aotearoa/New Zealand*. Palmerston North: Dunmore Press.

Bell, A. (2004a). 'Cultural vandalism and Pakeha politics of guilt and responsibility.' In P. Spoonley, C. Macpherson and D. Pearson (eds), *Tangata, Tangata: The Changing Ethnic Contours of New Zealand*. Southbank, Victoria: Dunmore Press.

Bell, A. (2004b). 'Relating Maori and Pakeha: The Politics of Indigenous and Settler Identities.' Doctoral thesis. Palmerston North: Massey University.

Billig, M. (1995). *Banal Nationalism*. London: Sage.

Billig, M., Condor, S., Edwards, D., Gane, M., Middleton, D., Radley, A. (1988). *Ideological Dilemmas: A Social Psychology of Everyday Thinking*. London: Sage.

Bourdieu, P. (1986). 'The forms of capital.' In J. Richardson (ed.), *Handbook of Theory and Research for the Sociology of Education*. New York: Greenwood Press.

Cain, V., Kingston, R. (2003). 'Investigating the role of racial/ethnic bias in health outcomes.' *American Journal of Public Health*, 93.

Chakraborty, A., McKenzie, K. (2002). 'Does racial discrimination cause mental illness?' *British Journal of Psychiatry*, 180: 475–7.

Corner, J. (1995). *Television Form and Public Address*. London: Edward Arnold.

Cunningham, C., Durie, M. (2005). 'Te rerenga hauora.' In K. Dew and P. Davis (eds), *Health and Society in Aotearoa New Zealand*. Melbourne: Oxford University Press.

Dressler, W. (1990). 'Lifestyle stress and blood pressure in a southern black community.' *Psychosomatic Medicine* 52: 182–98.

Durie, M. (2000). 'Maori health: Key determinants for the next twenty-five years.' *Pacific Health Dialog*, 7: 6–11.

Durie, M. (2004). *Effective interventions with young Maori: The Aotearoa reality* (Seminar Notes). New Plymouth: Compass Seminars.

Edley, N. (2001). 'Analysing masculinity: interpretative repertoires, ideological dilemmas and subject positions.' In M. Wetherell, S. Taylor and S. Yates (eds), *Discourse as Data: A Guide for Analysis*. London: Sage.

Fairclough, N. (1993). 'Critical discourse analysis and the marketisation of public discourse: the universities.' *Discourse and Society*, 4: 133–68.

Fairclough, N. (1995). *Media Discourse*. London: Arnold.

Fish, S. (1980). *Is There a Text in this Class?: The Authority of Interpretive Communities*. Cambridge, MA: Harvard University Press.

Fitzgerald, E. (2004). 'Development since the 1984 Hui Taumata.' In P. Spoonley, C. Macpherson and D. Pearson (eds), *Tangata Tangata: The Changing Ethnic Contours of New Zealand*. Melbourne: Thomson.

Foster, B.J. (2005). 'Featherston, Dr Isaac Earl.' In *Te Ara – The Encyclopedia of New Zealand*, edited by A.H. McLintock, originally published in 1966, updated 11 July 2005. http://www.TeAra.govt.nz/1966/F/FeatherstoneDrIsaacEarl/en

Foucault, M. (1972). *Archeology of Knowledge*. London: Tavistock.

Gavey, N. (1989). 'Feminist poststructuralism and discourse analysis: contributions to a feminist psychology.' *Psychology of Women Quarterly*, 13: 459–76.

Gee, G. (2002). 'A multilevel analysis of the relationship between institutional and individual racial discrimination and health status.' *American Journal of Public Health*, 92: 615–24.

Gergen, K. (1990). 'Towards a postmodern psychology.' *Humanistic Psychologist*, 18: 23–34.

Goldberg, D. (1993). *Racist Culture, Philosophy and the Politics of Meaning*. Oxford: Blackwell.

Hall, S. (2001). 'The spectacle of the other.' In M. Wetherell, S. Taylor and S. Yates (eds), *Discourse Theory and Practice: A Reader*. London: Sage, pp. 324–44.

Harrell, J., Hall, S. and Taliaferro, J. (2003). 'Physiological responses to racism and discrimination: An assessment of the evidence.' *American Journal of Public Health*, 93: 243–9.

Hattie, J. (2003). Presentation at Knowledge Wave 2003 – the Leadership Forum, University of Auckland, February. http://www.knowledgewave.org.nz/forum_2003/speeches/Hattie%20J.pdf

Herman, E., Chomsky, N. (1988). *Manufacturing Consent: The Political Economy of the Mass Media*. New York: Pantheon Books.

Hodgetts, D., Chamberlain, K. (2003). 'Narrativity and the mediation of the health reform agenda.' *Sociology of Health and Illness*, 25: 553–70.

Hodgetts, D., Masters, B., Roberston, N. (2004). 'Media coverage of "Decades of Disparity" in ethnic mortality in Aotearoa.' *Journal of Community Applied Social Psychology*, 14: 1–18.

Howden-Chapman, P. (2005). 'Unequal socioeconomic determinants, unequal health.' In K. Dew and P. Davis (eds), *Health and Society in Aotearoa New Zealand*. Melbourne: Oxford University Press.

James, S. (2003). 'Confronting the moral economy of US racial/ethnic disparities.' *American Journal of Public Health*, 93: 189.

James, S., LaCroix, A., Kleinbaum, D., Strogatz, D. (1984). 'John Henryism and blood pressure among black men: The role of occupational stressors.' *Journal of Behavioural Medicine*, 7: 258–75.

Karlsen, S. and Nazroo, J. (2003). 'Relation between racial discrimination, social class, and health among ethnic minority groups.' *American Journal of Public Health*, 92: 624–31.

Kelsey, J. (2002). *At the Crossroads: Three Essays*. Wellington: Bridget Williams Books.

King, M. (2003). *The Penguin History of New Zealand*. Auckland: Penguin Books.

Krieger, N. (1990). 'Racial and gender discrimination: Risk factors for high blood pressure.' *Social Science and Medicine*, 30: 1273–81.

Krieger, N. (2003). 'Does racism harm health? Did child abuse exist before 1962? On explicit questions, critical science, and current controversies: An ecosocial perspective.' *American Journal of Public Health*, 93: 194–200.

Krieger, N., Sidney, S. (1996). 'Racial discrimination and blood pressure: the CARDIA Study of young Black and White adults.' *American Journal of Public Health*, 86: 1370–8.

LaVeist, T. (2003). 'Racial segregation and longevity among African-Americans: An individual-level analysis.' *Health Services Research*, 38: 1719–33.

Marcovitch, H. (2005). 'What's new this month in BMJ Journals.' *BMJ*, 330: 116.

Marmot, M. and Wilkinson, R. (eds) (1999). *Social Determinants of Health*. New York: Oxford University Press.

McCreanor, T. (1989). 'Talking about race.' In H. Yensen, K. Hague and T. McCreanor (eds), *Honouring the Treaty: An Introduction for Pakeha to the Treaty of Waitangi*. Auckland: Penguin Books, pp. 90–118.

McCreanor, T. (1993a). 'Mimiwhangata: Media reliance on Pakeha commonsense in interpretations of Maori actions.' *Sites*, 26: 79–90.

McCreanor, T. (1993b). 'Pakeha ideology of Maori performance: A discourse analytic approach to the construction of educational failure in Aotearoa/New Zealand.' *Folia Linguistica*, 27: 293–314.

McCreanor, T. (1993c). 'Settling grievances to deny sovereignty: Trade good for the year 2000.' *Sites*, 27: 45–73.

McCreanor, T. (1996). '"Why strengthen the city when the enemy has poisoned the well?" An essay on anti-homosexual discourse in New Zealand.' *Journal of Homosexuality*, 31: 75–105.

McCreanor, T. (1997). 'When racism stepped ashore: Antecedents of anti-Maori discourse in New Zealand.' *New Zealand Journal of Psychology*, 23: 43–57.

McCreanor, T. (2005). '"Sticks and stones may break my bones ...": talking Pakeha identities.' In J. Liu, T. McCreanor, T. McIntosh and T. Teaiwa (eds), *New Zealand Identities: Departures and Destinations*. Wellington: Victoria University Press, pp. 52–68.

McGregor, J., Comrie, M. (1995). *Balance and Fairness in Broadcasting News 1985–1994*. Palmerston North: Massey University.

McKendrick, J., Thorpe, M. (1998). 'The legacy of colonisation: Trauma, loss and psychological distress among aboriginal people.' *Grief Matters*, 1: 4–8.

McKenzie, K. (2003). 'Racism and health: Antiracism is an important health issue.' (editorial). *British Medical Journal*, 326: 65–66.

Moewaka Barnes, A., Gregory, M., McCreanor, T., Nairn, R., Pega, F., Rankine, J. (2005). *Media and Te Tiriti o Waitangi*. Auckland: Kupu Taea.

Moser, T. (1888). *Mahoe Leaves: Being a Selection of Sketches of New Zealand and its Inhabitants, and Other Matters Concerning Them* (2nd edn). Wanganui: H.I. Jones and Son.

Nairn, R. (1999). 'Does the use of psychiatrists as sources improve media depictions of mental illness? A pilot study.' *Australia and New Zealand Journal of Psychiatry*, 33: 583–9.

Nairn, R., McCreanor, T. (1990). 'Sensitivity and insensitivity: an imbalance in Pakeha accounts of Maori/Pakeha relations.' *Journal of Language and Social Psychology*, 9: 293–308.

Nairn, R., McCreanor, T. (1991). 'Race talk and common sense: Patterns in Pakeha discourse on Maori/Pakeha relations in New Zealand.' *Journal of Language and Social Psychology*, 10: 245–62.

Nairn, R., Pega, F., McCreanor, T., Rankine, J., Barnes, A. (2006). 'Media, racism and public health psychology.' *Journal of Health Psychology*, 11(2): 183–96.

Nazroo, J. (2003). 'The structuring of ethnic inequalities in health: Economic position, racial discrimination, and racism.' *American Journal of Public Health*, 93: 277–85.

Orange, C. (1987). *The Treaty of Waitangi*. Wellington: Allen and Unwin.

Pember Reeves, W. (1899). *Aotearoa, Land of the Long White Cloud*. London: Horace Marshall & Son.

Pew Foundation (2005). 'What is civic journalism?' Retrieved 7 November 2005. http://www.pewcenter.org/doingcj/

Phelan, M., Stradins, L., Morrison, S. (2001). 'Physical health of people with severe mental illness.' *British Medical Journal*, 322: 443–44.

Pomare, E. (1980). *Maori Standards of Health: A Study of the Period 1955–1975*. Wellington: Medical Research Council of New Zealand.

Pomare, E., Keefe Ormsby, V., Ormsby, C., *et al.* (1995). *Hauora: Maori Standards of Health III: A Study of the Years 1970–1991*. Wellington: Eru Pomare Maori Research Centre.

Potter, J., Wetherell, M. (1987). *Discourse Analysis and Social Psychology: Beyond Attitudes and Behaviour*. London: Sage.

Raeburn, J. (2001). 'Community approaches to mental health promotion.' *International Journal of Mental Health Promotion*, 3: 13–19.

Ramsden, I., Spoonley, P. (1993). 'The cultural safety debate in nursing education in Aotearoa.' *New Zealand Annual Review of Education*, 4.

Rankine, J., McCreanor, T. (2004). 'Colonial coverage: media reporting of a bicultural health research partnership.' *Journalism*, 5: 5–29.

Reid, P., Cram, F. (2005). 'Connecting health, people and country in Aotearoa New Zealand.' In K. Dew and P. Davis (eds), *Health and Society in Aotearoa New Zealand*. New York: Oxford University Press.

Rose, G. (1992). *The Strategy of Preventive Medicine*. Oxford: Oxford University Press.

Rosenberg, W. (2002). 'News media ownership: How New Zealand is foreign-dominated.' *Pacific Journalism Review*, 8: 59–95.

Sanson, A., Augoustinos, M., Gridley, H., Kyrios, M., Reser, J., Turner, C. (1998). 'Racism and prejudice: An Australian Psychological Society position paper.' *Australian Psychologist*, 33: 161–82.

Scammell, M., Semetko, H. (2000). *The Media, Journalism and Democracy*. Aldershot: Ashgate.

Sharp, A. (1990). *Justice and the Maori: The Philosophy and Practice of Maori Claims in New Zealand Since the 1970s*. Auckland: Oxford University Press.

Sinclair, A. (1977). *The Savage: A History of Misunderstanding*. London: Weidenfeld and Nicolson.

Smith, L. (1999). *Decolonizing Methodologies: Research and Indigenous Peoples*. Dunedin: University of Otago Press/London: Zed Books.

Smith, L., Simon, J. (2001). *A Civilising Mission?: Perceptions and Representations of the Native Schools System*. Auckland: Auckland University Press.

Snedden, P. (2005). *Pakeha and the Treaty; Why it's Our Treaty Too*. Auckland: Random House.

Spoonley, P., Pearson, D., Macpherson, C. (eds) (1991). *Nga Take: Ethnic Relations and Racism in Aotearoa/New Zealand*. Palmerston North: Dunmore Press.

Sutherland, I. (ed.) (1940). *The Maori People Today: A General Survey*. Wellington: New Zealand Institute of International Affairs & the New Zealand Council for Educational Research.

Swan, P. (1998). 'Grief and health.' *Grief Matters*, 1: 9–11.

US Department of Health and Human Services (2002). 'Mental Health: Culture, Race, and Ethnicity, A Supplement to Mental Health: A Report of the Surgeon General.' Retrieved 5 November 2005. http://www.mentalhealth.samhsa.gov/cre/toc.asp

van Dijk, T. (1993). 'Principles of critical discourse analysis.' *Discourse and Society*, 4: 249–83.

Walker, R. (1990a). *Ka Whawhai Tonu Matou*. Auckland: Penguin.

Walker, R. (1990b). 'The role of the press in defining Pakeha perceptions of the Maori.' In P. Spoonley and W. Hirsh (eds), *Between the Lines: Racism and the New Zealand Media*. Auckland: Heinemann Reed, pp. 37–46.

Wallack, L. (2003). 'The role of mass media in creating social capital: A new direction for public health.' In R. Hofrichter (ed.), *Health and Social Justice*. Danvers, MA: John Wiley, pp. 594–625.

Wetherell, M., Potter, J. (1992). *Mapping the Language of Racism: Discourse and the Legitimation of Exploitation*. New York: Harvester Wheatsheaf.

Williams, D. (1999). 'Race, socioeconomic status, and health. The added effects of racism and discrimination.' *Annals of the New York Academy of Sciences*, 896: 173–88.

Williams, D., Neighbors, H., Jackson, J. (2003). 'Racial/ethnic discrimination and health: Findings from community studies.' *American Journal of Public Health*, 93: 200–9.

Williams, D., Williams-Morris, D. (2000). 'Racism and mental health: The African-American experience.' *Ethnicity and Health*, 5: 243–68.

Wilson, G. (1990). 'New Zealand journalists: Only partly professional.' In P. Spoonley and W. Hirsh (eds), *Between the Lines: Racism and the New Zealand Media*. Auckland: Heinemann Reed, pp. 47–55.

Witten, K., Kearns, R., Lewis, N., Coster, H., McCreanor, T. (2003). 'Educational restructuring from a community viewpoint: A case study from Invercargill, New Zealand.' *Environment and Planning C: Government and Policy*, 21: 203–23.

World Health Organization (1986). *Ottawa Charter for Health Promotion*, Geneva: WHO. Retrieved 14 June 2006, http://www.who.int/hpr/NPH/docs/ottawa_charter_hp.pdf

# Chapter 7

Adler, N.E. (2003). 'Looking beyond the borders of the health sector: The socio-economic determinants of health.' In E.R. Rubin and S.L. Schappert (eds), *Meeting Health Needs in the 21st Century*. Washington, DC: Association of Academic Health Centres, pp. 14–27.

Department of Labour (1994). *An Analysis of the Dynamics of the Registered Unemployed: Exit Probabilities and Repeat Spells*. Wellington: Department of Labour.

Dixon, S. (1998). 'Growth in the dispersion of earnings: 1984–1997.' *Labour Market Bulletin*, pp. 71–107.

Easton, B.H. (1996). 'Income distribution.' In B. Silverstone, A. Bollard, & R. Lattimore (eds), *A Study of Economic Reform: The Case of New Zealand*. Amsterdam: Elsevier, pp. 101–38.

Easton, B.H. (1999). 'What has happened in New Zealand to income distribution and poverty levels.' In S. Shaver & P. Saunders (eds), *Social*

*Policy for the 21st Century: Justice and Responsibility*, Vol 2. Sydney: SPRC, pp. 55–66.

Easton, B.H. (2002). Validation and the Health and Household Economy Project, Paper to the Wellington Health Economists Group, http://www.eastonbh.ac.nz/article229.html

Easton, B.H., Ballantyne, S. (2002). *The Economic and Health Status of Households*.Wellington: School of Medicine.

Idler, E., Levanthal, H., McLaughlin, J., Leventhal, E. (2004). 'In sickness but not in health: Self-ratings, identity, and mortality.' *Journal of Health and Social Behavior*, 45: 336–56.

Kawachi, I., Kennedy, B.P. (2002). *The Health of Nations: Why Inequality Is Harmful to Your Health*. New York: New Press.

Perry, B. (2005). *Social Report Indicators for Low Incomes and Inequality: Update from the 2004 Household Economic Survey*. Wellington: Ministry of Social Development.

Royal Commission of Inquiry on Social Security in New Zealand (1972). *Social Security in New Zealand, Report of the Royal Commission*. Wellington: Government Printer.

Sapolsky, R. (2004). *Why Zebras Don't Get Ulcers: A Guide to Stress, Stress Related Diseases and Coping*. New York: W.H. Freeman.

Sapolsky, R. (2005). 'Sick of Poverty.' *Scientific American*, December 2005, pp. 72–9.

Wilkinson, R. (2005). *The Impact of Inequality: How to Make Sick Societies Healthier*. New York: New Press.

Wilkinson, R., Marmot, M. (1998). *The Social Determinants of Health: The Solid Facts*. Copenhagen: WHO Regional Office for Europe.

# Chapter 8

Blair, T. (1999). 'Beveridge revisited: A welfare state for the 21st century.' In R. Walker (ed.), *Ending Child Poverty*. Bristol: Policy Press.

Child Poverty Action Group. (2000). *CPA Submission to the Government on Extending the Child Tax Credit to All Children*. Auckland: Child Poverty Action Group, www.cpag.org.nz

Child Poverty Action Group. (2002). *Challenging the Child Tax Credit. Case Taken to the Human Rights Commission under the Human Rights Act*. Auckland: Child Poverty Action Group, www.cpag.org.nz

Child Poverty Action Group. (2003). *Our Children. The Priority for Policy* (2nd edn).Auckland: Child Poverty Action Group.

Dornan, P. (ed.) (2004). *Ending Child Poverty by 2020. Five years on*. London: Child Poverty Action Group.

Duncan, G. (2006). *Income and child wellbeing* (No. 34). Dublin: Economic and Social Research Institute, http://wwwesri.ie

McLeod, R. (2001). *The Issues* (Tax review 2001). Wellington: New Zealand Government.

Ministry of Social Development. (2002). *New Zealand's Agenda for Children.* Wellington: Ministry of Social Development, http://wwwmsd.govt.nz/documents/publications

Ministry of Social Development. (2004). *New Zealand Families Today.* Wellington: Ministry of Social Development.

Mowbray, M. (2001). *Distributions and Disparity. New Zealand Household Incomes.* Wellington: Ministry of Social Policy.

Nolan, P. (2004a). *Family and Employment Tax Credits in Five Anglo-American countries.* Wellington: School of Government, Victoria University of Wellington.

Nolan, P. (2004b). 'When work does not pay: Family structures and poverty traps in New Zealand's social security system.' Paper presented at the New Zealand Association of Economists Conference, Wellington.

O'Brien, M. (2005). *Workfare: Not Fair for Kids? A Review of Compulsory Work Policies and Their Effects on Children.* Auckland: Child Poverty Action Group, http://www.cpag.org.nz

Perry, B. (2004). 'Working for families: The impact on child poverty.' *Journal of Social Policy, Ministry of Social Development,* 22, 19–54.

Perry, B. (2005). *Social Report Indicators for Low Incomes and Inequality: Update from the 2004 Household Economic Survey,* http://www.msd.govt.nz/work-areas/cross-sectorial-work/indicators-for-low-incomes-and-inequality.html

Shaw, C., Blakely, T., Crampton, P., Atkinson, J. (2005). 'The contribution of causes of death to socioeconomic inequalities in child mortality: New Zealand 1981–1999.' *New Zealand Medical Journal,* 118(1227): 1–11.

St John, S. (2004). Financial assistance for the young: 1986–2008, Discussion paper series No. 25, Department of Economics, University of Auckland.

St John, S., Craig, D. (2004). *Cut Price Kids: Does the 2004 'Working for Families' Budget Work for Children?* Auckland: Child Poverty Action Group.

St John, S., Dale, C., O'Brien, M., Blaiklock, A., Milne, S. (2001). *Our Children: The Priority for Policy.* Auckland: Child Poverty Action Group.

Stephens, R., Gray, D., Preston, D. (1996). 'New Zealand.' In J.B.T. Eardley, J. Ditch, I. Gough and P. Whiteford (eds), *Social Assistance in OECD Countries: Country Reports* (Vol. Report No. 47). London: Department of Social Security Research, HMSO, pp. 289–316.

Wynd, D. (2005). *Hard to Swallow.* Auckland: Child Poverty Action Group. http://www.cpag.org.nz

## Chapter 9

Acheson D. (1988). *Public Health in England: A Report to the Committee of Inquiry into the Future Development of the Public Health Function.* London: HMSO.

Auckland District Health Board (2002). *Strategic Plan.* http://www.adhb.govt.

nz/downloads/reports/2002/adhb_strategic_planmarch6.pdf. Accessed 14 June 2006.

Cardiac Inherited Diseases Group (2005). http://www.cidg.org/webcontent/Default.aspx?tabid=75. Accessed 14 June 2006.

European Commission (2002). *Public Health. Rare Diseases*. http://ec.europa.eu/health/ph_threats/non_com/rare_diseases_en.htm. Accessed 14 June 2006.

Ministry of Health (2002a). 'He Korowai Oranga – Māori Health Strategy.' Accessed 14 June 2006.

Ministry of Health (2002b). *A Framework for Public Health Action*. Wellington: Ministry of Health.

Ministry of Health (2005). *Newborn Metabolic Screening Programme*. Wellington: Ministry of Health. Accessed 14 June 2006.

Ministry of Health (2006a). 'The National Screening Unit. Universal Newborn Hearing Screening.' Update 6 March 2006. Wellington: Ministry of Health. Accessed 14 June 2006.

Ministry of Health (2006b). 'Directorate information.' http://www.moh.govt.nz/moh.nsf/wpg_index/About-moh-structure-directorates#1. Accessed 14 June 2006.

National Advisory Committee on Health and Disability (2003). *Molecular Genetic Testing in New Zealand: A Report of the National Advisory Committee on Health and Disability*. Wellington: Ministry of Health. http://www.nhc.govt.nz/publications/Genetics/GeneticTestingNZ.pdf. Accessed 14 June 2006.

National Health Committee (1998). *The Social, Cultural and Economic Determinants of Health in New Zealand: Action to Improve Health*. Wellington: Ministry of Health.

National Organisation for Rare Disorders (NORD) (2006). http://www.rarediseases.org/info/about.html. Accessed 14 June 2006.

New Zealand Food Safety Authority/Ministry of Health (2004). *Reducing Neural Tube Defects in New Zealand*. Consultation document No 2/04. July 2004. Wellington: New Zealand Food Safety Authority/Ministry of Health.

New Zealand Organisation for Rare Disorders (2007). 'International Genetic Alliance. Policy statement on the need for improved information, diagnosis, clinical care and treatment for rare diseases.' http://www.nzord.org.nz/internal.asp?CategoryID=100009&SubCatID=100066&ArticleID=100198. Accessed 21 June 2007.

Office of Rare Diseases (2006). 'The Genetic and Rare Diseases Information Centre.' http://rarediseases.info.nih/gov/html/resources/gard_brochure.html. Accessed 14 June 2006.

Stone P., Austin D. (2006). 'Assessment of Antenatal Screening for Down Syndrome in New Zealand. Auckland UniServices.' http://www.moh.govt.nz/moh.nsf/pagesmh/3455/$File/assessment-antenatal-screening-down-syndrome.pdf. Accessed 14 June 2006.

World Health Organization (1986). *Ottawa Charter for Health Promotion*, Geneva: WHO. http://www.who.int/hpr/NPH/docs/ottawa_charter_hp.pdf. Accessed 14 June 2006.

# Chapter 10

*Acknowledgements*
I would like to acknowledge the insightful contributions of Jon Foley, New
Zealand Ministry of Health, and the thoughtful comments provided by the
editors on earlier drafts of the chapter.

*References*
Advisory Committee on Hospital Board Funding (1980). *The Equitable
Distribution of Finance to Hospital Boards Report by the Advisory
Committee on Hospital Board Funding to the Minister of Health, The Hon
George F. Gair.* Wellington: Department of Health.
Advisory Committee on Hospital Board Funding (1986). *Report on the Review
of the Population-Based Method of Funding Hospital Boards, A report to
the Minister of Health, the Hon Dr M.E.R. Bassett.* Wellington: Advisory
Committee on Hospital Board Funding.
Beauchamp, T., Childress, J. (1989). *Principles of Biomedical Ethics.* New
York: Oxford University Press.
Birch, S., Chambers, S. (1993). 'To each according to need: a community-
based approach to allocating health care resources.' *Canadian Medical
Association Journal,* 149: 607–12.
Blakely, T., Kiro, C., Woodward, A. (2002). 'Unlocking the numerator-
denominator bias. II: adjustments to mortality rates by ethnicity and
deprivation during 1991–94. The New Zealand Census-Mortality Study.'
*New Zealand Medical Journal,* 115: 43–8.
Busse, R. (2004). 'Disease management programs in Germany's statutory
health insurance system.' *Health Affairs,* 23: 56–67.
Campbell, G. (2005). 'Change of tack.' *New Zealand Listener,* July 23–29,
14–17.
Crampton, P., Dowell, A., Woodward, A. (2001). 'Third sector primary care
for vulnerable populations.' *Social Science and Medicine,* 53: 1491–1502.
Crampton, P., Sutton, F., Foley, J. (2002). 'Capitation funding of primary care
services: principles and prospects.' *New Zealand Medical Journal,* 115:
27–4.
Eyles, J., Birch, S., Chambers, S., Hurley, J., Hutchinson, B. (1991). 'A
needs-based methodology for allocating health care resources in Ontario,
Canada: Development and application.' *Social Science and Medicine,* 33:
489–500.
Gribben, B. (1996), 'The community services card and utilisation of general
practitioner services.' *New Zealand Medical Journal,* 109: 103–5.
Hefford, M., Crampton, P., Foley, J. (2005). 'Reducing health disparities
through primary care reform: The New Zealand experiment.' *Health
Policy,* 72: 9–23.
Holohan, J., Rangarajan, S., Schirmer, M. (1999). *Medicaid Managed Care
Payment Methods and Capitation Rates: Results of a National Survey.
Occasional Paper no. 26,* Washington DC: The Urban Institute.

HURA Research Alliance, McLeod, D., Cormack, D., Love, T., Salmond, C., Robson, B., Dowell, A., Howard, M., Crampton, P., Ramage, S. (2006). 'Ethnicity, socioeconomic deprivation and consultation rates in New Zealand general practice.' *Journal of Health Services Research & Policy*, 11: 141–9.

Hutchison, B., Hurley, J., Birch, S., Lomas, J., Walter, S., Eyles, J., Stratford-Devai, F. (2000). 'Needs-based primary medical care capitation: Development and evaluation of alternative approaches.' *Health Care Management Science*, 3: 89–99.

King, A. (2001). *The Primary Health Care Strategy*. Wellington: Ministry of Health.

Kronick, R., Gilmer, T., Freyfus, T., Lee, L. (2000). 'Improving Health-based Payment for Medicaid Beneficiaries: CDPS.' *Health Care Financing Review*, 21: 29–63.

Majeed, A., Bindman, A., Weiner, J. (2001). 'Use of risk assessment in setting budgets and measuring performance in primary care II: Advantages, disadvantages, and practicalities.' *British Medical Journal*, 323: 607–10.

Medical Services Committee (1948). *Report of the Medical Services Committee*. Wellington: Medical Services Committee.

Ministry of Health (2005). *The Annual Report 2004/05 Including The Health and Independence Report: Annual Report for the year ended 30 June 2005: Director General of Health's Annual Report on the State of Public Health 2005*. Wellington: Ministry of Health.

Ministry of Health and the University of Otago (2006). *Decades of Disparity III: Overlapping Ethnic and Socio-economic Mortality Inequalities in New Zealand, 1981–1999*. Wellington: Ministry of Health.

Oliver, W. (1988). 'Social Policy in New Zealand: An Historical Overview.' *The April Report Volume 1, New Zealand Today, Report of The Royal Commission on Social Policy*. Wellington: The Royal Commission on Social Policy.

Pearce, N., Pōmare, E., Marshall, S., Borman, B. (1993). 'Mortality and social class in Māori and non-Māori New Zealand men: changes between 1975–7 and 1985–7.' *New Zealand Medical Journal*, 106: 193–6.

Pope, G., Ellis, R., Ash, A., Liu, C., Ayanian, J., Bates, D., Burstin, H., Iezzoni, L., Ingber, M. (2000). 'Principal inpatient diagnostic cost group model for Medicare risk adjustment.' *Health Care Financing Review*, 21: 93–118.

Rice, N., Smith, P. (2001). 'Capitation and risk adjustment in health care financing: An international progress report.' *Milbank Quarterly*, 79: 81–113.

Royal Commission of Inquiry on Social Security in New Zealand (1972). *Social Security in New Zealand, Report of the Royal Commission*. Wellington: Government Printer.

Salmond, C., Crampton, P. (2000). 'Deprivation and Health.' In P. Howden-Chapman and M. Tobias (eds), *Social Inequalities in Health: New Zealand 1999*. Wellington: Ministry of Health.

Salmond, C., Crampton, P. (2002). 'NZDep2001 Index of Deprivation.' Wellington: Department of Public Health, Wellington School of Medicine and Health Sciences.

Scott, K., Marwick, J., Crampton, P. (2003). 'Utilisation of general practitioner services in New Zealand and its relationship with income, ethnicity and government subsidy.' *Health Services Management Research*, 16: 45-55.

Shen, Y., Ellis, R. (2002). 'How Profitable is Risk Selection? A Comparison of Four Risk Adjustment Models.' *Health Economics*, 11: 165–74.

Starfield, B. (1998). *Primary Care, Balancing Health Needs, Services, and Technology*. New York: Oxford University Press.

Sutton, F. (2000). *Population-based Funding for Primary Care: Method and Results, a Report Prepared for the Health Funding Authority*. Wellington: Health Funding Authority.

van den Ven, W., van Vliet, R., Lamers, L. (2004). 'Health adjusted premium subsidies in the Netherlands.' *Health Affairs*, 23: 45–55.

van Doorslaer, E., Masseria, C., Koolman, X. (2005). 'Inequalities in access to medical care by income in developed countries.' *Canadian Medical Association Journal*, 174: 177–83.

Weiner, J., Abrams, C. (2001). *The Johns Hopkins ACG Case-Mix System, Documentation & Application Manual*. Baltimore: The Johns Hopkins University Bloomberg School of Public Health.

Weiner, J., Starfield, B., Lieberman, R. (1992). 'Johns Hopkins ambulatory care groups: a case-mix system for UR, QA, and capitation adjustment.' *HMO Practice*, 6: 13–19.

Zhao, Y., Ash, A., Ellis, R., Slaughter, J. (2002). 'Disease Burden Profiles: An Emerging Tool for Managing Managed Care.' *Health Care Management Science*, 5: 211–19.

# Chapter 11

Bunker, J.P., Frazier, H.S., Mosteller, F. (1994). 'Improving health: Measuring the effects of medical care.' *Milbank Quarterly*, 72: 225–8.

Hart, J.T. (1971). 'The Inverse Care Law.' *The Lancet*, 1: 405–12.

Health Services Research Centre, Te Rōpū Rangahau Hauora a Eru Pōmare (2001). National Demonstration integrated Care Pilot Projects. Overview Report. Final Evaluation Report (unpublished).

Howden-Chapman, P., Tobias, M. *et al.* (eds) (2000). *Social Inequalities in Health: New Zealand 1999*. Wellington: Ministry of Health.

King, A. (2000). *The New Zealand Health Strategy*. Wellington: Ministry of Health.

King, A. (2001). *The Primary Health Care Strategy*. Wellington: Ministry of Health.

King, A, Turia, T. (2002). *He Korowai Oranga. Maori Health Strategy*. Wellington: Ministry of Health.

Lantz, P.M., House, J.S., Lepkowski, J.M., *et al.* (1998). 'Socio-economic factors, health behaviours, and mortality: Results from a nationally representative prospective study of US adults.' *Journal of the American Medical Association*, 279: 1703–8.

Ministry of Health (1999). *Our Health, Our Future: The Health of New Zealanders, 1999*. Wellington: Ministry of Health.

Ministry of Health (2003a). *Healthy Eating – Healthy Action. Oranga Kai – Oranga Pumau. A strategic Framework*. Wellington: Ministry of Health.

Ministry of Health (2003b). *Evaluation of Culturally Appropriate Smoking Cessation Programme for Māori Women and their Whānau. Aukati Kai Paioa 2000*. Wellington: Ministry of Health.

Ministry of Health (2004). *General Practice Fees Information. A Summary of Key Findings from Five Reports*. Wellington: Ministry of Health.

National Advisory Committee on Health and Disability (1998). *The Social, Cultural and Economic Determinants of Health in New Zealand: Action to Improve Health*. Wellington: National Advisory Committee on Health and Disability.

National Health Committee (2000). *Improving Health for New Zealanders by Investing in Primary Health Care*. Wellington: National Health Committee.

Shi, L. (1997). 'Health care spending, delivery, and outcome in developed countries: A cross-national comparison.' *American Journal of Medical Quality*, 12: 83–93.

Shi, L., Starfield, B., Kennedy, B., *et al*. (1999). 'Income inequality, primary care, and health indicators.' *Journal of Family Practice*, 48: 275–84.

Starfield, B. (1994). 'Is primary care essential?' *The Lancet*, 344: 1129–33.

Te Puni Kōkiri (1998). *Progress Towards Closing Social and Economic Gaps Between Māori and Non-Māori. A Report to the Minister of Māori Affairs*. Wellington: Te Puni Kōkiri.

World Health Organization (1978). *Primary Health Care. Report of the International Conference on Primary Health Care, Alma Ata., USSR*. Geneva: WHO.

World Health Organization (2002). *The World Health Report 2002. Reducing Risks, Promoting Healthy Lives*. Geneva: WHO.

## Chapter 12

Ambrose, P., Nicholson, P. (2004). Appendix 1 – Income 'before housing costs' – an incomplete measure of poverty. *Memorandum to the Prime Minister on Minimum Income Standards*. London: Zacchaeus Trust, pp. 11–15.

Baker, M., McNicholas, A., Garrett, N., Fafphm, N., Stewart J., Koberstein V., Lennon, D. (2000). 'Household crowding a major risk factor for meningococcal disease in Auckland children.' *Paediatric Infectious Disease Journal*, 19: 983–90.

Baker, M., Milosevic, J., Blakely, T., Howden-Chapman, P. (2004). 'Housing, crowding and health.' In P. Howden-Chapman and P. Carroll (eds), *Housing & Health: Research, Policy and Innovation*. Wellington: Steele Roberts, pp. 57–69.

Baker, M., Zhang, J. (2005). 'Housing, Crowding and Health Study: Characteristics of cohort members and selected hospitalisation events: February 2003 to June 2005.' *Housing and Health Research Programme Reports*. Wellington: University of Otago.

Baker, M., Das, D., Venugopal, K., Howden-Chapman, P. (forthcoming). 'Household crowding and tuberculosis in New Zealand.' *Journal of Epidemiology and Community Health.*

Belgrave, M., (2004). 'Needs and the state: Evolving social policy in New Zealand history.' In B. Dalley and M. Tennant (eds), *Past Judgement: Social Policy in New Zealand History.* Dunedin: University of Otago Press, pp. 22–38.

Bierre,S.,Cunningham,C.,Cunningham,M.,Baker,M.,Robinson,J.,Kennedy, M. *et al.* (2004). *A Healthy Housing Index: A Collaborative Approach to Measuring Housing Condition.* The Second WHO International Housing and Health Symposium, Vilnius, Lithuania, Geneva: WHO.

Bierre S., Howden-Chapman, P., *et al.* (2007). 'Insititutional challenges in addressing healthy low-cost housing for all: Learning from past policy.' *Social Policy Journal of New Zealand*, 30: 42–64.

Blakely, T., Woodward, A., Pearce, N., Salmond, C., Kiro, C., Davis, P. (2002). 'Socio-cconomic factors and mortality among 25–64 year olds followed from 1991 to 1994: The New Zealand Census-Mortality Study.' *New Zealand Medical Journal*, 115: 93–7.

Chapman, R., Howden-Chapman. P., O'Dea, D., Viggers, H., Kennedy, M. (Submitted for publication). 'Retrofitting houses with insulation: cost-benefit analysis of a randomised community trial.'

Davie, G. (2004). *The Seasons of 'Six Feet Under': Trends and Determinants of Excess Winter Mortality in New Zealand from 1980 to 2000.* Melbourne: Department of Biostatistics, University of Melbourne.

Davis, P., Howden-Chapman, P. (1996). 'Translating research findings into health policy.' *Social Science and Medicine*, 43(5): 865–72.

Dew, K., Carroll, P. (2007). 'Public Health and CAM perspectives: An exploration of overlap, contrast and dissonance.' In J. Adams (ed.), *Researching Complementary and Alternative Medicine.* London and New York: Routledge.

Dickens, P., Duncan, S., Goodwin, M., Gray, F. (1985). *Housing, States and Localities.* London: Methuen.

Ferguson, G. (1994). *Building the New Zealand Dream.* Palmerston North: Dunmore Press.

Garrett, M., Abramson, M., Hooper, B., Rayment, P., Strasser, R., Hooper, M. (1998). 'Indoor environment risk factors for respiratory health in children.' *Indoor Air*, 8: 236–43.

Graham, H. (ed.) (2001). *Understanding Health Inequalities.* Buckingham: Open University Press.

Gregory, A. (2006). 'State tenants excluded from new neighbourhoods.' *NZ Herald.* 12 January 2006.

Harris, R., Tobias, M., Jeffreys, M., Waldegrave, K., Karlsen, S., Nazroo, J. (2006). 'Effects of self-reported reacial discrimination and deprivation on Maori health and inequalities in New Zealand: Cross sectional study.' *The Lancet*, 367: 2005–9.

Healy, J.D. (2004). *Housing, Fuel Poverty and Health: A Pan-European analysis*. Aldershot: Ashgate.

Howden-Chapman, P. (2004). 'Housing standards: A glossary of housing and health.' *Journal of Epidemiology and Community Health*, 58: 162–8.

Howden-Chapman, P., Buchanan, S., Baker, M. (Submitted for publication). 'The impact of research on policy: Two housing case studies.' *Social Science and Medicine*.

Howden-Chapman, P., Crane, J., Baker, M., Cunningham, C., Matheson, A. (2004). 'Reducing health inequality through improving housing: He Kainga Oranga/ Housing & Health Research Programme.' In P. Howden-Chapman and P. Carroll (eds), *Housing & Health: Research, Policy and Innovation*. Wellington: Steele Roberts, pp. 83–92.

Howden-Chapman, P., Crane, J., Matheson, A., Viggers, H., Cunningham, M., Blakely, T. *et al.* (2005). 'Retrofitting houses with insulation to reduce health inequalities: aims and methods of a clustered, randomised trial in community settings.' *Social Science and Medicine*, 61(12): 2600–2610.

Howden-Chapman, P., Matheson A., Viggers, H., Crane, J., Cunningham, M., Blakely, T., *et al* (2007). 'Retrofitting houses with insulation to reduce health inequalities: results of a clustered randomised trial in a community setting.' *British Medical Journal*, 334: 460–4

Howden-Chapman, P., Pene, G., Crane, J., Green, R., Iupati, L., Prior, I., *et al*. (2000). 'Open houses and closed rooms: Tokelau housing in New Zealand.' *Health Educ. Behav.*, 27(3): 351–62.

Howden-Chapman, P., Pierse, N., Nicholls, S., Cunningham, M., Phipps, R., Boulic, M. *et al*. (2007). *The Housing, Heating and Health Study: Preliminary Results May 2007*. www.wnmeds.ac.nz/healthyhousing.html.

Howden-Chapman, P., Saville-Smith, K., Crane, J., Wilson, N. (2005). 'Risk factors for mould.' *Indoor Air*, 15: 469–76.

Howden-Chapman, P., Tobias, M. (eds) (2000). *Social Inequalities in Health: New Zealand 1999*. Wellington: Ministry of Health.

Howden-Chapman, P., Wilson, N. (2000). 'Housing and health.' In P. Howden-Chapman & M. Tobias (eds), *Social Inequalities in Health: New Zealand 1999*. Wellington: Ministry of Health, pp. 133–46.

Isaacs, N. (2005). 'HEEP delivers national results.' *Build*, Oct/Nov, 98–99.

Israel, B., Schulz, A., Parker, E., Becker, A. (1998). 'Review of community-based participatory research: Assessing partnership approaches to improving public health.' *Annual Review of Public Health*, 19: 173–202.

Keall, M., Baker, M., Howden-Chapman, P., Cunningham, M. 'Association between the number of home injury hazards and home injury.' *Accident Analysis and Prevention*, (in press).

Kuila, J. (1993). 'Integrating Government Assistance for Accommodation.' *Social Policy Journal of New Zealand*, 1: 44–50.

Le Grand, J., Propper, C., Robinson, R. (1984). *Economics of Social Problems*. Basingstoke: Palgrave.

Lloyd, B. (2006). 'Fuel poverty in New Zealand.' *Social Policy Journal of New Zealand*, 27: 142–55.

MacDonald, J. (1986). *Racism and Rental Accommodation*. Auckland: New Zealand Office of the Race Relations Conciliator.

Maori Women's Housing Research Project (1991). '…*for the sake of decent shelter* …' Wellington: Housing Corporation of New Zealand.

Marsh, A., Gordon, D., Pantazis, C., Heslop, P. (2000). *Home Sweet Home? The Impact of Housing on Health*. Bristol: The Policy Press.

Matheson, A., Howden-Chapman, P., Dew, K. (2005). 'Engaging communities to reduce inequalities in health: why partnership?' *Social Policy Journal of New Zealand*, 26: 1–16.

McClure, M. (2004). 'A badge of poverty or a symbol of citizenship? Needs, rights and social security, 1935–2000.' In B. Dalley and M. Tennant (eds), *Past Judgement: Social Policy in New Zealand History*. Dunedin: University of Otago Press, pp. 140–55.

McNicholas, A., Lennon, D., Crampton, P., Howden-Chapman, P. (2000). 'Overcrowding and infectious diseases – when will we learn the lessons of our past?' *New Zealand Medical Journal*, 113(1121): 453–4.

Ministry of Health (2002). *Reducing Inequalities in Health*. Wellington: Ministry of Health.

Ministry of Social Development (2005). *The Social Report 2005*. Wellington: Ministry of Social Development.

Ministry of Social Policy (2005). http://www.beehive.govt.nz/breifings/socialpolicy/housing/3.cfm

Murphy, L. (1999). 'Housing Policy.' In J. Boston, P. Dalziel and S. St John (eds), *Redesigning the Welfare State in New Zealand*. Auckland: Oxford University Press, pp. 218–37.

Murphy, L., Kearns, R. (1994). 'Housing New Zealand Ltd: Privatisation by stealth.' *Environment and Planning*, 26: 623–37.

Næss, Ø., Claussen, B., Davey Smith, G., Thelle, D. (2004). 'Cumulative deprivation and cause-specific mortality: A census-based study of mortality by housing-conditions over three decades.' *Journal of Epidemiology and Community Health*, 58: 599–603.

National Housing Commission (1988). *Housing New Zealand: Provision and Policy at the Crossroads*. Wellington: National Housing Commission.

New Zealand Treasury (1984). *Economic Management*. Wellington: Government Printer.

New Zealand Treasury (1987). *Government Management*. Wellington: Government Printer.

New Zealand Treasury (1990). *Briefing to the Incoming Government*. Wellington: Government Printer.

O'Dea, D., Chapman, R., Howden-Chapman, P. 'Willingness to pay for the financial, comfort, and health benefits of home insulation.' (Submitted for publication.)

Oliver, W.H. (1988). 'Social Policy in New Zealand: An Historical Overview.'

*Royal Commission on Social Policy, The April Report*. Wellington: Government Printer.

Pene, G., Howden-Chapman, P., Crane, J., Viggers, H., Southwick, M., Iupati, L. (2002). *Housing and Health in the Tokelau Community*. Wellington: Housing and Health Research Programme.

Robinson, B. (2005). *A Home I Could Own: What Do Low Income Families Want from Housing?* Wellington: Salvation Army.

Rose, G. (1992). *The Strategy of Preventive Medicine*. Oxford: Oxford University Press.

Shrader, B. (2005). *We Call it Home: A History of State Housing in New Zealand*. Auckland: Reed.

Spoonley, P. (1975). Prospects for the Niuean Community in Auckland: The Role of Gate Keeper Groups in Migrant Adaptation. MA Thesis, Department of Geography, University of Otago, Dunedin.

Statistics New Zealand (2007). http://www.stats.govt.nz/census/2006-census-data/quickstats-about-housing-revised.htm?page=para009Master

Tennant, M. (2004). 'History and social policy: Perspectives from the past.' In B. Dalley and M. Tennant (eds), *Past Judgement: Social Policy in New Zealand History*. Dunedin: University of Otago Press, pp. 9–22.

Thomson, D. (1991). *Selfish Generations? The Ageing of New Zealand's Welfare State*. Wellington: Bridget Willams Books.

Thomson, G., Wilson, N., Howden-Chapman, P. (2005). 'Smoky homes: A review of the exposure and effects of secondhand smoke in New Zealand homes.' *New Zealand Medical Journal*, 118: 213.

Thomson, H., Petticrew, M., Morrison, D. (2001). 'Health effects of housing improvement: Systematic review of intervention studies.' *British Medical Journal*, 323: 187–90.

Thorns, D.H. (1988). 'Housing Issues.' *Royal Commission on Social Policy April 1988*, III. Wellington: Government Printer, pp. 5–25.

Thorns, D.H. (2000). 'Housing policy in the 1990s – New Zealand a decade of change.' *Housing Studies*, 15(1): 129–38.

Trlin, A.D. (1977). 'State housing shelter and welfare in suburbia.' In A.D. Trlin (ed), *Social Welfare and New Zealand Society*. Wellington: Methuen Publications, pp. 106–31.

Turner, R., Baker, M., Milosevic, J. (2004). *Housing, Crowding and Health Study: Characteristics of Applicants and Tenants for the Period February 2003 to July 2004*. Housing and Health Research Programme. Wellington: Department of Health and University of Otago.

Waldegrave, C., Love, C., Stuart, C. (2000). 'Urban Maori responses to changes in state housing provision.' *Social Policy Journal of New Zealand*, 14: 114–29.

Widmer, S. (2006). *Assessing the Relation Between Housing Policy, Overcrowding, and Infectious Diseases in New Zealand*. Housing and Health Research Programme, Wellington: Department of Health and University of Otago.

World Health Organization (1987). *Health Impact of Low Indoor Temperatures: Report on a WHO Meeting, Copenhagen, 11–14 November, 1985.* Copenhagen: WHO.

# Chapter 13

*Acknowledgements*

I would like to thank the workshop and research participants for their role in building an understanding about these equity tools. I would also like to thank my colleagues at the Wellington School of Medicine and Health Sciences and the Ministry of Health for collaborating with me on the work presented in this chapter.

Ajwani, S., Blakely, T., *et al.* (2003). *Decades of Disparity: Ethnic Mortality Trends in New Zealand 1980–1999.* Wellington: Ministry of Health and University of Otago.

Blakely, T., Fawcett, J., *et al.* (2005). *Decades of Disparity II: Socioeconomic Mortality Trends in New Zealand, 1981–1999.* Wellington: Ministry of Health and University of Otago.

Bro Taf Authority (2000). *Planning for Positive Impact: Health Inequalities Impact Assessment Tool.* Cardiff: Bro Taf Authority.

Carroll, C., Howden-Chapman, P., *et al.* (2004). *Tackling Inequalities: Moving Theory to Action.* Wellington: Ministry of Health.

European Centre for Health Policy (1999). *Health Impact Assessment: Main Concepts and Suggested Approach.* Brussels: European Centre for Health Policy.

Graham, H. (ed.) (2001). *Understanding Health Inequalities.* Buckingham: Open University Press.

Howden-Chapman, P., Tobias, M. (eds) (2000). *Social Inequalities in Health: New Zealand 1999.* Wellington: Ministry of Health.

Jones, C. (1999). *Maori-Pakeha Health Disparities: Can Treaty Settlements Reverse the Impacts of Racism?* Wellington: Ian Axford Fellowships Office.

Jones, C. (2000). 'Levels of racism: a theoretic framework and a gardener's tale.' *American Journal of Public Health*, 90: 1212–5.

Krieger, N. (2001). 'A glossary for social epidemiology.' *Journal of Epidemiology and Community Health*, 55: 693–700.

Lykes, M., Banuazizi, A., *et al.* (eds) (1996). *Myths About the Powerless: Contesting Social Inequalities.* Philadelphia: Temple University Press.

Mackenbach, J.P., Bakker, M.J., *et al.* (2002). 'Strategies to reduce socioeconomic inequalities in health.' In J.P. Mackenbach (ed.), *Reducing Socioeconomic Inequalities in Health: A European Perspective.* London: Routledge, pp. 25–49.

March, J., Olsen, J. (1984). 'The new institutionalism: organizational factors in political life.' *American Political Science Review*, 78: 734–49.

Martin, H. (2002). *TUHA-NZ a Treaty Understanding of Hauora in Aotearoa-New Zealand: An understanding about the application of te Tiriti o Waitangi in health promotion practice in Aotearoa-New Zealand*. Auckland: Health Promotion Forum of New Zealand.

Minister for Disability Issues (2001). *The New Zealand Disability Strategy: Making a World of Difference: Whakanui Oranga*. Wellington: Ministry of Health.

Ministry of Health (2000). *The New Zealand Health Strategy*. Wellington: Ministry of Health.

Ministry of Health (2002). *He Korowai Oranga: Māori health strategy*. Wellington: Ministry of Health.

Ministry of Health (2002). *Reducing Inequalities in Health*. Wellington: Ministry of Health.

Ministry of Health, Public Health Consultancy, *et al*. (2004). *A Health Equity Assessment Tool. Amended by the Ministry of Health 2004*. Wellington: Ministry of Health.

National Health Committee (1998). *The Social, Cultural and Economic Determinants of Health in New Zealand: Action to Improve Health*. Wellington: National Health Committee. Public Health Consultancy, Te Rōpū Rangahau Hauora a Eru Pōmare.

Public Health Advisory Committee (2005). *A Guide to Health Impact Assessment: A Policy Tool for New Zealand* (2nd edn). Wellington: National Advisory Committee on Health and Disability.

Ryan, W. (1971). *Blaming the Victim*. New York: Pantheon.

Signal, L. (2002). 'Tacking inequalities through health promotion action.' *Health Promotion Forum of New Zealand Newsletter*, 56: 10.

Signal, L., Martin, J. (2005). *A Review of the Use of Equity Tools in the New Zealand Health Sector*. Wellington: Wellington School of Medicine and Health Sciences.

Signal, L.N., Durham, G. (2000). 'Health impact assessment in the New Zealand policy context.' *Social Policy Journal of New Zealand*, 15: 11–26.

South East Health (2003). *Four Steps Towards Equity: A Tool for Health Promotion Practice*. Sydney: Health Promotion Service, South East Health.

Woodward, A., Kawachi, I. (2000). 'Why reduce health inequalities?' *Journal of Epidemiology and Community Health*, 54: 923–9.

## Chapter 14

Bullen, C. (1999). *Action on Housing and Health in Otara: A Report to the National Health Committee*. Wellington: Ministry of Health.

Cheer, T. (2000). Discounting Health and Healthcare in Low Income Households in Otara. MA Thesis, Dept of Geography, University of Auckland.

Cheer, T., Kearns, R., Murphy, L. (2002). 'Housing policy, poverty and culture: "discounting decisions" among Pacific peoples in Auckland.' *New Zealand Environment and Planning C : Government and Policy*, 20(4): 497–516.

248 Understanding health inequalities in Aotearoa New Zealand

Community Forum (1977). Statement of Community Development Beliefs – Fiji Y.M.C.A Rural Workers.

Haigh, D. (2000). *Otara Health and Housing Campaign August 2000 Evaluation*. Auckland: Sidelines Ltd.

Housing New Zealand Corporation (2003). *Healthy Housing Development Programme*. Wellington: Housing New Zealand.

Howden-Chapman, P., Crane, J., Matheson, A., Viggers, H., *et al.* (2005). 'Retrofitting houses with insulation to reduce health inequalities: aims and methods of a clustered, randomised trial in community settings.' *Social Science and Medicine*, 61(12): 2600–10.

Johnson, A., James, O. (2001). *Our Home Our Place. Report on the Otara Housing Hui: Whaiora Marae March 2001*. Auckland: Otara Health Incorporated.

Lennon, M. (2003). 'Housing Provision in New Zealand.' In P. Howden-Chapman & P. Carroll (eds), *Housing and Health: Research, Policy and Innovation*. Wellington: Steele Roberts, pp. 70–3.

Mitchell, P. (1995). *The Otara Primary and Public Health Needs Asessment Report*. Auckland: North Health.

National Health Committee (1998). *The Social, Cultural and Economic Determinants of Health: Action to Improve Health*. Wellington: National Health Committee.

North Health (1995). *Primary Care Strategy*. Auckland: North Health.

Simmons, D., Weblemoe, T., Voyle, J., Prichard, A., Leakehe, L., Gatland, B. (1998). *Personal Barriers to Diabetic Care: Lessons from a Multiethnic Community in New Zealand*. Auckland: South Auckland Division of Clinical Science, Middlemore Hospital and University of Auckland.

World Health Organization (1986). *Ottawa Charter for Health Promotion*. WHO: Geneva. http://www.who.int/hpr/NPH/docs/ottawa_charter_hp.pdf. Accessed 14 June 2006.

# Chapter 15

*Acknowledgements*

This chapter is an acknowledgement of the work and dedication of those who contributed their reflections and stories and also of all the other people who dedicate their lives to improving the health of those who are outside the mainstream health system.